Caring for the
8 Truths to Prolong Your Career

Michael A. Sherbun, PhD, MHA, RN
Senior Director of Psychiatry
Cincinnati Children's Hospital
Cincinnati, Ohio

Founder, The Workplace Doctor
www.workplacedoc.com

JONES AND BARTLETT PUBLISHERS
Sudbury, Massachusetts
BOSTON   TORONTO   LONDON   SINGAPORE

World Headquarters

Jones and Bartlett Publishers
40 Tall Pine Drive
Sudbury, MA 01776
978-443-5000
info@jbpub.com
www.jbpub.com

Jones and Bartlett Publishers
Canada
6339 Ormindale Way
Mississauga, Ontario L5V 1J2
Canada

Jones and Bartlett Publishers
International
Barb House, Barb Mews
London W6 7PA
United Kingdom

Jones and Bartlett's books and products are available through most bookstores and online book-sellers. To contact Jones and Bartlett Publishers directly, call 800-832-0034, fax 978-443-8000, or visit our website www.jbpub.com.

Substantial discounts on bulk quantities of Jones and Bartlett's publications are available to cor-porations, professional associations, and other qualified organizations. For details and specific discount information, contact the special sales department at Jones and Bartlett via the above contact information or send an email to specialsales@jbpub.com.

Library of Congress Cataloging-in-Publication Data

Sherbun, Michael A.
  Caring for the caregiver : 8 truths to prolong your career / Michael A. Sherbun.—1st ed.
    p. cm.
  Includes bibliographical references.
  ISBN 0-7637-3080-7 (pbk. : alk. paper)
  1. Nurse and patient. 2. Nursing—Psychological aspects. 3. Caregivers—Psychology.
I. Title.
  RT86.3.S546 2006
  610.73'06'99—dc22

                                                                                    2005013172

Production Credits
Acquisitions Editor: Kevin Sullivan
Production Director: Amy Rose
Associate Editor: Amy Sibley
Associate Production Editor: Carolyn F. Rogers
Marketing Manager: Emily Ekle
Manufacturing and Inventory Coordinator: Amy Bacus
Composition: Auburn Associates, Inc.
Cover Design: Kristin Ohlin
Printing and Binding: Malloy, Inc.
Cover Printing: Malloy, Inc.

Printed in the United States of America
09 08 07 06 05   10 9 8 7 6 5 4 3 2 1

DEDICATION

To my mother, Dolores, for her strong spiritual beliefs and
persistent support of those less fortunate than herself
and
To my wife, Leslie, for her constant belief in and
support of me in pursuing this dream.

CONTENTS

INTRODUCTION

Welcome to *Caring for the Caregiver: 8 Truths to Prolong Your Career*. This book will be the first in a series of books designed to reconnect you to your work and teach you how to improve your emotional health. This unique approach is different because it is created for you. It is designed to address the specific work issues, stressors, and dynamics in your industry. Creating one book to address everyone's emotional health issues doesn't work. The specific issues you all face in your individual world are unique and different.

Caring for the Caregiver: 8 Truths to Prolong Your Career is dedicated to health care professionals. Their unique stressors and issues at work can be found in no other setting. This book uses true personal stories to outline the complicated work lives of health care professionals. Provided throughout the book are true and tested communication principles, a road map for guiding health care professionals in managing all types of personalities.

These techniques also provide a process to help you reconnect to yourself, a chance to create a new work experience. Somewhere along the line nurses and other health care professionals lost their way trying to remember why they entered this field and struggle to remain in it.

Understanding your reality and determining what you can and cannot control is the first step in beginning to reconnect with yourself. So many health care professionals continue to live each day in an unconscious state. They do not understand the connection between who they are and the world they create.

Through tools such as the Circle of Control, the Control Reaction Map, and the Success Steps model, health care professionals learn to understand the differences in everyone's personality. They understand that each interaction is an opportunity to place others "in control." They understand the connection between their own unique self (Circle of Control) and their responses to others. Because of this understanding, their defenses are lowered and their need to win all the time is diminished. This creates a different experience in their lives. They do not perceive their stressors in the same way. They are more peaceful and happy.

With the guidelines for reducing stress and conflict, health care professionals learn to create a plan that moves them closer to wellness and avoids an all-too-common experience in this field: burnout.

I hope this book will provide for you a sense of peace and enlightenment. In an area where you did not perceive change could occur, it can. In an area that you believed would always have stress, you don't have to. Even if the external factors affecting your work and field change only minimally, your perception of them will change greatly. Use this book to create a new experience and a new you.

TRUTH #1:

UNDERSTANDING YOUR REALITY

What Your Peers Are Saying About Being a Nurse or Health Care Worker Today

Whatever we focus on becomes our idea of reality.

—Anthony Robbins

Welcome to *Caring for the Caregiver: 8 Truths to Prolong Your Career*. These eight truths are intended to teach you how to look at your world differently and create a new experience. This is like no other self-help book you have read. It was written specifically for nurses and other health care professionals *by* a health care professional. The stories are real and designed to let you know what your colleagues across the country are experiencing. The techniques are unique and immediately applicable. They will provide for you a road map on how to manage all the personality types you interact with in your health care setting. They will reconnect you to your career and yourself, and in the end you will be happier. You will understand how to create a different experience. It all begins with the first truth, understanding the realities of health care today and how it affects your world.

Do these situations sound familiar to you?

Your patient is anxious, the family is upset. It seems that no matter what you do, it isn't enough to please them. The complaining is nonstop. You find yourself avoiding them as much as possible.

Suddenly, the two patients you were caring for in the ICU have become three, with the third being a new admission. No help is offered. This isn't the first time. You're overwhelmed.

For the most part you get along with your co-workers. There are two staff members who complain continuously, but they are the first ones to avoid work. No one says anything to them, and the dynamic never changes. Enjoying your work becomes harder every day.

Your supervisor micro-manages everything on the unit. Your input is asked for but never used. It feels like an effort in futility. Someone finally addressed this with her, and she denies this style. You feel stifled with no room to grow.

Why We Chose to Be Health Care Professionals

You were drawn to this profession because you wanted to make a difference, you wanted to serve people, you wanted to make them well, or you wanted to help them find their own path to wellness. You were drawn to this profession for very noble reasons.

Unfortunately, the norm for health care professionals now is to be dissatisfied, disgruntled, and maybe even bitter about their experiences. I don't know how or why we have arrived at this point, but it is clear that a problem exists, and it appears that it has gotten worse over the years.

For 20 years I have been a nurse, an administrator, and now an author and public speaker. I love my work. At the same time, after 20 years, I realized how hard it is to watch caring, enthusiastic professionals become unhappy about their work, burned out, and, in some cases, even bitter and vengeful. Truthfully, I just got tired of it. As a professional committed to healing, I concluded that it does not have to be this way and that I needed to do something. So I began trying to understand how we arrived at this point and what we can do about it.

In my search to understand, I had the privilege of speaking with over 1,000 nurses and other health care professionals. In all of these conversations, I was struck by the enthusiasm and conviction these people showed for their chosen careers. I was also struck by how little control they felt they had—over their work and over their lives. Why was that? How could this dichotomy exist? How could they feel very strongly about what they were doing and confident about their skills while at the same time feel helpless and discouraged with their careers and, in some cases, their lives?

> **Over 60% of nurses entered the profession of nursing because of a calling to help others.**

I gained an enormous amount of insight through these interviews. One of the most interesting insights was that over 60% of you entered the profession of nursing because of a calling to help others. There was a sense of connection to taking care of others and healing. However, there was a great deal of dissatisfaction. It became quite clear that much of the dissatisfaction had to do with the lack of connection to your patients, the hospital, and your peers. You told me it became harder to remember why you entered this profession because it was harder to see the results. If nurses are dissatisfied with their connection to their patients, their workplace, and their peers, is it any wonder that the rates of turnover, burnout, and unhappiness are so high?

This intrigued me and, truthfully, has become my passion. I did not set out to write a book, just to make a difference. The more people I spoke with, the more passionate I became, and the clearer it became that I *had* to write this book to assist my fellow health care workers. I realized that we can change our experience of the world in which we live but that it takes diligent effort, a great deal of self-management, the support of others, and a commitment to ourselves and our peers that matches or exceeds our original commitment to this profession.

Dealing with life and death on a daily basis and constant change in the health care environment does not have to lead to a sense of loss of control and frustration. It does not have to affect your perception of who you are at work or in your family life.

It is time for a new approach to teaching health care professionals how to regain control of their lives. That's what you'll find in this book in an easy to use, immediately applicable way. Not only will you learn the eight truths to reconnect and ignite your enthusiasm at work and at home, but you will also experience the stories of nurses throughout the country who share your struggles. Their stories will connect with you, inspire you, and then demonstrate how you can apply these tools to help you achieve control in your own life.

You will hear stories about new graduates who left their careers in panic because of the overwhelming nature of the dynamics of our industry. You will hear a story of a nurse with over 10 years of critical care experience who was loved by all of her patients until one of her patients decided not to cooperate, leaving her frustrated and second-guessing her own skills. You will hear of a nurse manager who accepted her first management assignment only to see her love of the profession and staff turn into a bitter and frustrating experience. You will learn about a unit clerk who misinterpreted interactions among her co-workers and began a long and disruptive battle against them. You will read about nurses with various personality struggles telling of those struggles, and you will also hear an inspiring story of a nurse who almost gave up on her profession, her marriage, and her life but who, by using the principles described in this book, regained control of herself, her family, and her profession.

This book is not about identifying ways to attract nurses. It is not a recruitment strategy book. It is not a guide to avoiding the nursing shortage. It is not about trying to convince you that you should or should not stay in this profession. What this book is about is you. It will help you rediscover your passion for caring, serving, making a difference, and healing. It will allow you to reconnect with yourself, your job, and your family. It is through this reconnection that you regain your circle of control and recreate success and passion for yourself.

It is time to rekindle the spirit that is inside you and to reignite your career and the love of yourself. Welcome to *Caring for the Caregiver*.

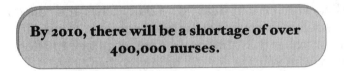

By 2010, there will be a shortage of over 400,000 nurses.

This first truth in *Caring for the Caregiver* was written for the purpose of providing you with an accurate picture of your reality, your reality being the current situation for nurses and other health care professionals, responses from health care professionals to these changes, and the realities of patient care and the changes that have occurred as a result of insurance guidelines, regulatory guidelines, and economic well-being of health care institutions. Understanding the context in which you work and all the factors influencing your experience builds the foundation for taking care of the caregiver.

A Unique Time in History

There has never been a time like this in the history of nursing. According to the American Hospital Association, we will have a shortage of over 400,000 nurses by 2020. They also report that 126,000 nurses are needed *today* to fill vacancies and that 75% of all hospital vacancies are for nurses. These startling statistics have been the primary catalyst reshaping our nursing profession. It has driven how we practice, how we relate to our peers, and it has become the motivation behind our administrative strategies.

You know these numbers and, more importantly, you have experienced the effects of this shortage. Your staff-to-patient ratio has increased, and the mix of nursing staff to aides, assistants, and other health care personnel has shifted dramatically. The result of all these changes is that you are more removed from the patient, thus altering the patient's care and experience. In addition, when you are further from providing the type of patient care you came into this industry for, it affects your satisfaction deeply. Your connection to your patients has been diminished. This is part of your reality.

Janette Erickson and Brenda Nevidjon, authors of *Nursing Shortage and Solutions for the Short and Long Term* (*Online Journal of Issues in Nursing*, January 31, 2001), report that the shortage we are experiencing today is different from past shortages and that we can expect it to worsen during the next decade as more nurses retire. They identify the key differences from the previous shortage as the following:

1. the age of nurses
2. general shortages in ancillary professionals and support labor
3. global nature of the shortage
4. impact of managed care

Approximately one third of the nursing workforce is over 50 years of age, and the average age of full-time nursing faculty is 49. A study published in the July 2000 issue of the *Journal of the American Medical Association* predicts that 40% of nurses will be 50 years or older by 2010.

What does this mean?

As nurses age and retire, there will be an even greater demand, a demand for nurses and on the time nurses have available for each patient and task, further diminishing connections to patients.

Erickson and Nevidjon (2001) further report that, "The fundamental changes in how patients are cared for in a managed care environment are compounding the shortage." Patients are staying in the hospital for shorter lengths of time. This, coupled with the need for more acute care in ambulatory and home settings, increases the demand for experienced, highly skilled nurses. This trend of sicker patients being treated with decreasing lengths of stays creates an increasingly stressful environment for nurses. There is an increased concern for nurses as a result of higher acuity, but the decreased length of stay presents an increased amount of work—and paperwork—for the same amount of staff. For example, a 12-bed med-surge unit with an average length of stay of 10 days produces 36 admissions per month. The same unit with an average length of stay of 5 days produces 72 admissions per month. The same number of nurses and other health care personnel manages the increase of 36 patients per month, and the staffing ratio is not adjusted, but the workload to complete admissions and discharges is greatly increased.

One nurse I interviewed stated that what she missed most over her 20-year career was hearing the words "thank you" from patients, families, and peers. She stated, "The whole environment has become harder to work in because everyone seems to be working at such a faster pace and (they) become easily frustrated by this. With all the changes that have occurred in health care, I am afraid we have lost the purpose of treating and helping patients and their families." This faster pace results in frustration and dissatisfaction, ultimately showing up as a lower tolerance level. This tone sets the pace and atmosphere for staff, patients, and families to have a poor experience.

This nurse is not alone. Eighty-five percent of the nurses I interviewed agreed that the changes in health care over the last 10 years have been dramatic enough to significantly alter the way they practice nursing. Nurses also report a significant decrease in job satisfaction. Many reported their jobs feeling more like an assembly line rather than a way of helping people heal in comfort. And, most unfortunately, most of these nurses, while keenly aware of their own dissatisfaction, are not seeing the impact of their care and feeling disconnected from patient care itself. In a report from Smith and Seccumbe in 1988, 611 registered nurses gave the following reasons for leaving their jobs:

- 93%: inadequate resources to do their jobs
- 88%: inadequate pay
- 86%: inadequate opportunity to develop their skills
- 81%: inadequate promotion prospects
- 81%: excessive workload
- 77%: inadequate career structure
- 75%: inflexible working hours

Coupled with these findings is the research completed in the 1980s regarding nursing satisfaction. J. P. Bush (1988), author of the article "Job Satisfaction, Powerlessness, and Loss of Control," defined nursing satisfaction from the psychological perspective. He stated, "The perception that one's job fulfills or allows the fulfillment of one's important job values, providing and to the degree that those values are congruent with one's needs." Butler and Parsons (1989), authors of the article "Hospital Perception of Job Satisfaction," emphasized workplace factors such as recognition of achievement, adequate staffing, appreciation, autonomy, child-care facilities, and quality patient care.

> **When nurses are not able to care for their patients in a way that matches their values, they leave.**

What this research demonstrates is that when nurses don't have adequate resources to do their jobs, aren't given the opportunity and time to develop their skills, have an excessive workload, don't feel appreciated, and aren't able to care for their patients in a way that matches their values, they will leave. And when they leave, not only does it affect the individual patients they were treating, it affects all the remaining nurses and health care professionals. In fact, it affects the entire industry. What does it cost to replace a nurse? Estimates for replacing a nurse range from $60,000 to $100,000. This does not include the effects of decreased morale and patient safety among those left behind.

Several authors in the 1990s added to what was identified in the 1980s when they defined what satisfaction means to nurses. According to Waite, Buchan, and Thomas (1989), authors of "Nurses In and Out of Work," patient care is fundamental to nurse satisfaction—fundamental, not just something nurses like to do. They measured their satisfaction based on the ability to give good patient care. In 1998, McKenna published "Editorials: The Professional Cleansing of Nurses," which supported the position that nurse satisfaction is based on quality patient care. "The quality and continuity of patient care, as well as patient outcomes, are improved when there are a sufficient number of qualified nurses working in a unit able to offer direct hands on patient care."

Most recently, the American Nurses Association reports the following satisfaction results from their survey in 2001. These results are startling but accurate, and they paint a clear picture of the reality for the caregiver today.

- 56% report direct patient care time has decreased.
- Overwhelming number of nurses have experienced "an increased patient care load," resulting in a dramatic decrease in the quality of patient care.
- 75% of nurses surveyed felt the quality of nursing care has declined in the last two years.
- #1 reason—Inadequate staffing
- #2 reason—Decreased nurse satisfaction
- #3 reason—Delay in provider basic care
- 54% of nurses would NOT recommend the nursing profession as a career for their children or friends.

These are the realities of your world.

The research and trends from the 1980s until today are consistent. Nurses value quality patient care and their satisfaction is tied to this. When you evaluate these facts, it is not hard to understand the concerns many nurses have. External variables have contributed to nurses being disconnected from their patients. Factors affecting patient care have decreased nursing and health care satisfaction levels.

Now what? It appears overwhelming. How can you find happiness in your work with such dramatic changes? Is there even any point?

Yes there is. The first truth, understanding your reality, is crucial to achieving happiness at work because before you can effect change, you have to understand the variables that are affecting your work.

The standard way of dealing with dissatisfaction is nonproductive. In fact, it can be detrimental. You spend your energy on anger and frustration over situations that are beyond your control. You continue to feel out of control, which leads to increased levels of dissatisfaction. This can materialize in your interactions at work and at home. You find yourself complaining about situations at work at an increasing pace until you discover this is all you speak about with your co-workers. You bring this "style" home with you and begin the same cycle. This negative energy is of no use to you. It keeps you from experiencing joy and happiness. Even knowing this, you repeat the cycle over and over again. Why? It is what you know, but you have been misguided. Continuing along this path will only lead to more dissatisfaction and unhappiness at work and within yourself, and, ultimately, you will continue to feel out of control.

You have an understanding of your reality. You understand the dynamics of health care as well as your specific profession. You know the reasons nurses stay and leave their jobs and, most importantly, you know they value quality patient care.

Understanding YOU

This book could focus on how to solve the nursing crisis. We could spend the next several chapters quoting the latest trends to attract and retain nurses, but that would do little to help caretakers take better care of themselves and begin to experience happiness in their work again. I am not saying this is not important work being done in our field, but despite all these efforts, these external factors will continue to be an issue. Understanding yourself and learning to manage your experience of these external events is essential to changing your experience.

You are still one person trying to do the job you chose to do and make a difference for patients and their families. You no longer can hope to find contentment and happiness waiting for the external factors to improve. If you try, you place your satisfaction and sense of self out of your control. Isn't that what many of you have been doing? You have become frustrated and angry about your career, blaming administrators, co-workers, and poor working conditions on your situation. In doing so, you may experience momentary relief, but it will not sustain you or help you take the best care of yourself in the long run.

You have to ask yourself, has this worked for me? I am assuming it has not and this is the reason you have chosen this book. Do not get me wrong. You cannot ignore all the external factors that affect your work environment, and we will address many of these in the upcoming truths. However, you will not solve the problem by using all your energies to attempt change. The realities of your workplace play only a small part in your search for happiness at work, and they make up the context in which you can create your own happiness: taking care of the caregiver.

Truth #2:

Determining Who You Are

Identifying Your Circle of Control

You can't solve a problem with the same mind that created it.

—Dr. Wayne Dwyer

Now that you understand the historical and contemporary context of your frustration, it is time to focus on you. With the second truth you will be reconnecting to your job and those around you through a conscious discovery of yourself. *Caring for the Caregiver* is not just about prolonging your career. It is about connecting with yourself, changing how you react to the world, and creating a new experience. For some of you, this is the first time you have done this. You have just reacted to life *and* avoided this, but I tell you it is worth looking at yourself, and it is necessary to changing your experience.

I am choosing to share with you a concept that focuses on the development of self. You see, there is so much discussion about how we can change the health care dynamics at the workplace to make ourselves happier and more fulfilled. These efforts are worthwhile, but it is not a path on which you will find happiness. Just think about it. If this were true, your sense of contentment at work and feelings of peace and joy would correlate fully with what the industry does or does not do. Rather, I choose to create a path that provides consistent and long-term happiness in your life. You all know as well as I do that it is very difficult to separate your personal and professional lives. In addition, the stressors that affect your external world are constant. As we set out to determine who you are, your Circle of Control, we do so with the idea that the first step in achieving happiness and real joy is getting to know yourself.

Determining your Circle of Control will help you feel a sense of peace and calmness in your life. By understanding your Circle of Control you are providing clarity to your life and making better choices about actions you can take. You will find that your external world makes sense and is less chaotic and stressful.

Why is this? What is it about these principles that can affect your life, that can create a sense of happiness for you when no external changes occur? The answer to this is "consciousness." So many people walk through life not understanding who they are. They continue to react to the external world and do not understand the connection between themselves and their actions. I wish I could tell you this was more complicated, but it is not. The first truth just requires people to become conscious of themselves or, better yet, conscious of their Circle of Control.

Creative Visualization, a national best-seller, says all of us have the ability to create our own experience. "To begin this process, the individual needs to understand who they are. True happiness and peace cannot occur until individuals have found introspection." As we discuss the eighth truth, "Creating Your Experience," we will refer to this book in greater detail. I highly recommend it.

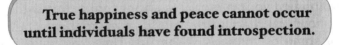

True happiness and peace cannot occur until individuals have found introspection.

So you can see, you have to be committed in this first truth to understanding who you are and to stop living life unconsciously and not understanding why there is a connection between who you are and your actions.

I have been referring to your Circle of Control in this truth. What is it? It is a picture of you. It includes three variables, each of which is essential. If you leave any variable unattended, it is like driving a car with the tires partially inflated or with a significant chunk missing. You might still get where you are going, but it would not be

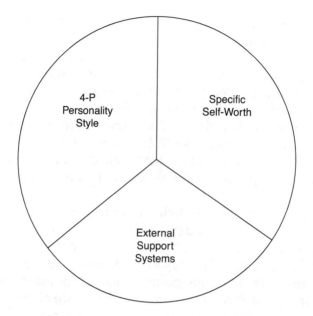

The Circle of Control

a smooth—or safe—ride. Without measuring each of the three variables that make up your map, you continue to react to the external aspects of your life in an unconscious style. Each of you has your own Circle of Control. It is a snapshot of you.

Circle of Control

The three variables of your Circle of Control are your 4-P Personality Style, your specific self-worth, and your external support systems.

All of us have a Circle of Control made up of these three variables, but most of us are unaware of them or how they affect our experience. In fact, we tend to deny our ability to manage our external world, instead playing the role of victim or martyr.

The problem with this is when you fail to manage or even acknowledge your Circle of Control, you also give up your chance at happiness, self-worth, and celebrating the difference you make to your patients. Not only is this unfair to you, it's unfair to your patients, their families, and your co-workers. By articulating who you are and how that relates to others, your specific self-worth and goals, and your support systems, you can begin to develop your Circle of Control, placing you in the driver's seat.

Determining your Circle of Control is not just a warm fuzzy step designed to make you feel good. The truth is that once you do this, you will immediately see your world change. You will not be able to view any of your problems in the same way, and you will begin to develop a sense of happiness that comes from being responsive to yourself in a whole new way. This initial inward step is essential to each of the subsequent steps for taking care of the caregiver. Do not gloss over this process. Give yourself the time and attention you deserve.

Here is the beauty of the Circle of Control: Each one is different. We all have our own unique personality style, support systems, and specific self-worth dynamics. Your circle will not look like anyone else's, and your circle today may not look like what you would have imagined 10 years ago. The point is not to compare circles with anyone else or form judgments. Instead, be aware of yours: how you can affect it and how you can maximize your strengths. A conscious understanding of your circle will help you manage issues that affect you in a more satisfying manner. This is the key. Most individuals allow life to happen to them and do not understand how to be aware of their own self and consciously decide how to react to the external world. I realize I have focussed on this point a great deal in this truth. However, I do this for a reason. I want you to understand the importance of this initial truth. You have to decide to be conscious and really see yourself.

4-P Personality Styles

Let's look at each aspect of the 4-P Personality Styles. Everyone has a style of his or her own. Although this is great because it contributes to the diversity of thoughts, ideas, and actions, it also poses some problems because we tend to forget that not everyone is like us. It is essential that we understand this. We do not have the same personality styles.

You have seen this throughout your life. Not all people respond the same way you do. Some people you connect with instantly, and with others, communication seems impossible. Some people you just "get," and others you never understand. Personality styles are more than just a party discussion. It helps you understand why you respond the way you do in all situations.

Have you taken personality tests? In my research I have found that most personality evaluations are too complicated and confusing, rendering them virtually useless as anything more than an interesting activity or game. To be a useful tool, a personality evaluation has to be something you can understand immediately and begin applying to your everyday interactions. For this reason I created my own tool called the 4-P Personality Style model. The purpose of this tool is to identify your predominant style. This model is easy to use,

Instructions for the 4-P Personality Style Evaluation

- In section 1, evaluate the characteristics in each of the six boxes and determine whether column A or column B best reflects your style. Circle A or B.
- Once you have completed this for all six boxes, please refer to section 2 to find the style of each one. Circle the style that equates to your choice of A or B for each box.
- In Section 3, total the number of each personality style that you identified and place that number under the appropriate personality style section.
- The majority of you will have a clearly identified personality style.
- Refer to characteristic grid on the following page to identify the specifics of your personality style.
- Some of you will have one or more categories with the same score. This means you possess characteristics of more than one personality style. However, you still have a dominant style. To determine this, first evaluate the characteristics grid on the following page and pay specific attention to the latest three categories—enjoys conflict, likes change, and works in a team. Does one style stand out for you? If it still does not, refer to page 27. During periods of stress, each personality style demonstrates very different behaviors; pointers direct, processors isolate and work, peacemakers care for others, and politicians socialize. This should finally clarify for your dominant style.

THE 4-P PERSONALITY STYLE EVALUATION

SECTION 1

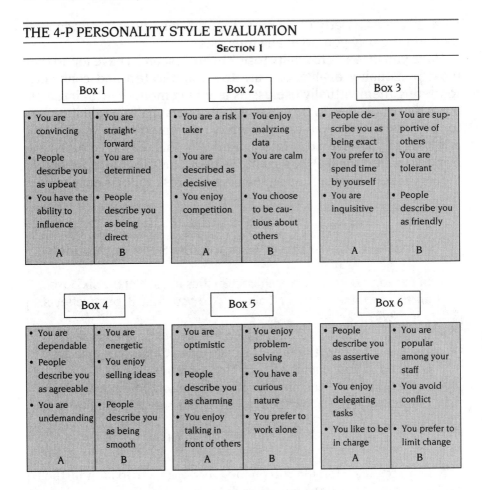

Box 1	
• You are convincing	• You are straight-forward
• People describe you as upbeat	• You are determined
• You have the ability to influence	• People describe you as being direct
A	B

Box 2	
• You are a risk taker	• You enjoy analyzing data
• You are described as decisive	• You are calm
• You enjoy competition	• You choose to be cautious about others
A	B

Box 3	
• People describe you as being exact	• You are supportive of others
• You prefer to spend time by yourself	• You are tolerant
• You are inquisitive	• People describe you as friendly
A	B

Box 4	
• You are dependable	• You are energetic
• People describe you as agreeable	• You enjoy selling ideas
• You are undemanding	• People describe you as being smooth
A	B

Box 5	
• You are optimistic	• You enjoy problem-solving
• People describe you as charming	• You have a curious nature
• You enjoy talking in front of others	• You prefer to work alone
A	B

Box 6	
• People describe you as assertive	• You are popular among your staff
• You enjoy delegating tasks	• You avoid conflict
• You like to be in charge	• You prefer to limit change
A	B

SECTION 2

Box 1 Style: A, Politician   B, Pointer
Box 2 Style: A, Pointer   B, Processor
Box 3 Style: A, Processor   B, Peacemaker
Box 4 Style: A, Peacemaker   B, Politician
Box 5 Style: A, Politician   B, Processor
Box 6 Style: A, Pointer   B, Peacemaker

SECTION 3

Total Number of Boxes Chosen			
Politician	Processor	Pointer	Peacemaker

easy to understand, and easy to start applying immediately, and there are no wrong answers or wrong personality styles.

Much of my work has been consulting to health care organizations because of staff conflicts. Invariably, I have found that all staff conflicts begin with a misinterpretation as a result of personality style. This misunderstanding leads to further misinterpretations and elevated conflicts. As you can imagine, this is a drain on vital energy and effort.

If, on the other hand, these staff members had spent time understanding their Circle of Control, they would have begun by determining each of their personality styles and then deciding how they could more effectively work together. Their energies would have been spent recognizing and appreciating individual differences and how to present information in a way everyone could understand it.

Each style has its own distinct characteristics; some of these characteristics you like, others you do not. You want to understand your style and the styles of those around you in order to guide you in your interactions. The purpose of this is greater understanding, not judging yourself or others for not being able to "do it better." Applying this information is how you begin to become conscious of your Circle of Control. You will find yourself watching how these various personality styles are expressed and how people with each style deal with the challenges of life in remarkably different ways. You will begin to see how easy it is to misinterpret or be misinterpreted without even realizing it.

We do not all think alike or problem solve in the same manner. That's the beauty of understanding the 4-P Personality Styles

CHARACTERISTIC GRID

	POINTER	POLITICIAN	PEACEMAKER	PROCESSOR
Characteristics	Straightforward	Convincing	Supportive	Exact
	Determined	Upbeat	Friendly	Loner
	Risk-taker	Influencial	Dependable	Inquisitive
	Decisive	Energetic	Agreeable	Analyzer
	Competitive	Smooth	Undemanding	Calm
	Assertive	Optimistic	Popular	Problem-solver
	Delegates	Charming	Conflict-avoider	Curious
Enjoys Conflict	YES!	NO	NO	NO
Likes Change	YES!	YES!	NO	NO
Works in a Team	NO	YES!	YES!	NO

model. Virtually all workplace conflict and stress stem from the lack of understanding of the different personality styles or the unwillingness to value each style. By understanding the various 4-P Personality Styles, you can and will avoid stress that stems from this lack of understanding. Having a fundamental knowledge of the four basic styles and how they think and process will save you energy, heartache, and burnout.

The 4-P Personality Styles are the *pointer*, the *politician*, the *processor*, and the *peacemaker*. Each of these will be explained in depth.

First, it is essential that you accept that there is no right or wrong personality style. The goal is to understand how you think, process, and interact with others to determine your own personal style. Secondly, you need to recognize that not everyone around you thinks your way. They are not wrong, just different. As a phrase from Neil Donald Walsch in his book, *Conversations with God: An Uncommon Dialogue*, stated, "Mine is not a better way, it is just a different one."

Let's begin determining your own Circle of Control by identifying your personality style. On the following page you will find a list of words you will rank according to how each best describes you. Once you have completed the evaluation, continue following directions to determine your personality style and specific style dynamics.

Have you identified your style? Have you looked at the grid to start to review the various characteristics for each personality style? Is it starting to make sense to you? You should find yourself starting to look back at your work and your personal life and see how these characteristics describe you. I have found in my seminars that this is a point where individuals begin to understand the Circle of Control. You really can relate to the idea that the individuals you interact with daily reflect one of these personality styles.

After 20 years working in health care, I began to realize and see these various personality styles at work. I began to identify the specific names within the 4-P Personality Style model. I did so after much assessment and assistance from many staff who were able to help me create this test. I was often called the "pointer" before these 4-P Personality Styles were developed because of my leadership abilities. There were numerous peacemakers on my staff who consistently provided a sense of calm in our chaotic world. We had quality-assurance and data-processing staff in our organization who reflected the processor personality style. Finally, our marketing and development colleagues, who were great at selling programs and raising money, helped us create the politician. The 4-P Personality Style model was created with you in mind, and after taking the test, I am sure you have already identified one of these styles that really reflects who you are.

The Pointer

Pointers are decisive and like to be in control. They are concerned about being in charge and getting results. They usually are strong leaders who are able to multitask and accomplish goals under pressure.

Pointers have limited tolerance for people who are inefficient or indecisive. They excel at transforming people and organizations because of their focus on results. Pointers enjoy delegating and are usually quite good at it. They are successful because of their ability to provide structure and stability. Pointers rise to the occasion during stressful times when decisions need to be made, particularly when they need to be made quickly. They welcome change and focus on the outcomes.

Let's look back at the characteristics of the pointers. They are described as being the boss and being in charge. They focus on the task at hand and the facts. They enjoy conflict, mainly because it provides them with an opportunity to achieve outcomes. They do not see change as a problem. They believe change is an opportunity to create a better outcome. When they are criticized, it is usually when they are working on a team. Others can sometimes see their directness and rather quick decision-making style as offensive. They may feel excluded.

We have talked about the traditional positions that pointers fill, but let's make sure we review and understand what they are. Managers, supervisors, and directors often are pointers. However, many charge nurses are placed in this role as well because of their ability to make quick decisions under pressure. This is what makes them successful. However, it can be also their downfall, because in their pursuit of the outcome, their consistency may be lacking, and this may be perceived as unfair by staff. Here are some quotes from staff describing their peers with the pointer style.

- "They are not afraid of anything."
- "They just jump right into any situation without hesitation."
- "He/she is too 'bossy' and not even my supervisor."

Here are some ways to understand staff who are pointers.

1. They look to lead staff, to be in charge, etc.
2. They like to manage staff projects.
3. They take the lead in problem-solving operational issues.
4. They may delegate duties more often to colleagues.

Can you think of some managers, supervisors, and other directors who have this pointer style? Can you identify stories in which decisions were made in which you do not feel that your opinion was even listened to or appreciated? If you have been in a situation like this, I want you to think of the outcome that occurred and how it affected your work and home life.

Supervisors, in general, are successful in this role. As we have identified, health care is becoming more complicated and stressful. Leaders who are pointers have the ability to manage this complexity and stress. It does not mean their style is perfect. Leaders with this style can frustrate many staff because of their "take charge" approach. Here is what staff have said about supervisors with this personality style.

- "All I have to do is ask, and it is taken care of."
- "It feels good to have a supervisor address the issues of the staff."
- "I want to be more involved, but every time I take on a project, he tells me how to do it."

Supervisors who are pointers

1. succeed at multitasking,
2. appear to manage more responsibilities than other directors/ managers/supervisors (and do not complain)
3. frequently delegate projects to employees,
4. will create a clear vision for a group and initiate change without hesitation.

The Politician

Simply put, these are your energetic, passionate people, often the life of the party or conversation. They thrive on recognition and are innovative and lively. They are also extremely spontaneous. Refer back to your characteristics grid. You will see the politician has an incredible ability to motivate others and can be a change agent for any program. They have the ability to brainstorm multiple ideas. They do not enjoy conflict, mainly because it is no fun. Conflict is not positive, it is not motivational, it can limit creativity. However, they do like change because change is an opportunity to be innovative. Change is an opportunity to create something new. Finally, they do enjoy working in a team, to a point. I say this because, usually, working in a team at some point requires individuals to manage all or a portion of a project, and politicians' attention to detail is an issue. This does not make them a popular team member when they don't complete their tasks. Are you starting to think about people that you work with who fit this personality style?

Health care workers with this style tend to be the ones who volunteer to organize events, and they are great on task forces and committees because of their brainstorming abilities. Health care professionals with this style gravitate to marketing, referral development, and customer service initiatives.

Politicians are great for morale. They always see the glass as half full, generating numerous ideas and making the atmosphere lighter and more fun. People of this style play a large role in staff retention and satisfaction. They are needed in work groups and problem-solving groups. Staff members, directors, and supervisors who have this personality style can be both rewarding and challenging to their peers and their employees.

As we stated earlier, having a fellow worker who is a politician can be wonderful. They can identify ways to better enjoy experiences at work. They often are the ones who like to initiate staff recognition programs, organize parties and get-togethers, and celebrate on a regular basis. Without a doubt, they are fun to have around.

However, it is difficult and frustrating working with politicians when they are unable to follow through with an agreed-upon task. Usually this is because of their lack of attention to detail. Here are some quotes that I have heard from staff members describing their peer politicians.

- "They are wonderful, but I feel like I am always picking up after them."
- "Sometimes they just appear to be unaware of what's happening around them especially when others of us need help."
- "They are always talking and not working."

These are just a few examples that can cause staff to be frustrated and angry at this personality style.

Staff who are politicians

1. are energetic and fun to be around,
2. unite staff through their energy and organized gatherings,
3. are solutions people; they brainstorm alternative methods,
4. help with change because of their positive nature.

In some circumstances, it can be wonderful to have a politician as your supervisor. Their ability to bring energy, excitement, and change to the unit, the program, and the hospital is wonderful. They have the ability to get everyone very excited about who they are and where they are going. They are not afraid to participate in direct care, leading by example, which is greatly supported by staff.

However, where a great deal of frustration (and I am speaking from experience) for staff exists is with the lack of follow-through and attention to detail. Despite the politicians' best efforts, they tend to move from project to project, leaving others with a sense of unfinished business and confusion.

Quotes that I have received from other individuals about politician supervisors are

- "She started off with a lot of energy, and now I don't know where she's going."
- "She has a lot of great ideas; I just don't see anything getting done."
- "I'm not sure what she expects from me. She keeps changing her mind all the time."

Supervisors who are politicians

1. create and provide innovative solutions,
2. are change agents to move past complacency,
3. motivate individual staff and teams.

The Peacemaker

The third style is the peacemaker, making up 60% of all health care staff. Peacemakers seek stability. They are well liked by their peers because of their focus on listening, teamwork, and follow-through. They seek agreement through conference and collaboration. Co-workers often describe them as reliable. It is fortunate to have peacemakers on your team because of their ability to calm the team and be a steady presence.

Let's take a look at the characteristics grid and understand more about the peacemaker. The one characteristic that does mark this personality style is the way these people strive for peace among everyone. They are extremely tolerant of the behavior of others. They are identified as very consistent individuals who provide a sense of stability. They do not enjoy conflict. The reason for this is that conflict results, in their minds, as instability among their co-workers, causing increased stress for them and their peers. As a result, they will then begin to work feverishly to meet with a number of their peers to identify an agreement on the issue. Their goal is to regain order. They do not like change because change results in conflict. However, they do love to work in a team, becoming the consummate team player attempting to assure that everyone is cared for and heard.

By far, the peacemakers are the most popular employees on the team. They will take the assignments that nobody else will take. They will assist in projects that are not desirable, and they will find the good in everyone despite what others may say.

However, where peacemakers have difficulties is in being taken advantage of. Because of their desire to create a team that is content and without conflict, they often give too much of themselves and begin to lose a sense of self, and in some instances, lose all boundaries. They have been described as co-dependent at times and need to be supported by their peers and supervisors to assure they take care of themselves as well as others.

Have you identified your peers that reflect this personality style? As stated earlier, this style accounts for the majority of health care workers.

Here is what staff are saying about peers with a peacemaker style.

- "She is the sweetest and kindest person I know."
- "There isn't anything she wouldn't do for me if I asked."
- "I worry about her. She is always taking care of others. I don't think she looks after herself."

Staff who are peacemakers

1. are concerned whether or not you are happy,
2. attempt to meet everyone's needs,
3. are well liked by all staff,
4. create peace and harmony for the team: "the buffer."

On the surface, it appears that working with or being supervised by a peacemaker would be very inviting and positive. However, there are certain characteristics that provide a challenge for individuals working with this personality style in both a supervisory as well as a peer role.

Because of their need to please and the need to provide or develop a sense of peace among their staff, they often promise more than they can possibly deliver. In their need and desire to please everyone (which is impossible), they become increasingly frustrated. Conflict naturally arises because someone will be unhappy, and the peacemaker manager is unable to achieve agreement among all the staff. This just further promotes their discontent in the management position and quite often peacemakers in these positions end up leaving health care organizations as a result of burnout and frustration.

Here is what staff say about supervisors with a peacemaker style.

- "They are very supportive of me and the team."
- "She does not seem to be herself. I think management is getting to her."
- "She is trying to please everyone. There is no way she can."

Supervisors who are peacemakers

1. want to create a truly healthy and supportive environment,
2. attempt to meet each staff member's needs,
3. avoid conflict and attempt to minimize concerns and problems.

The Processor

The processor's focus is on accuracy. Processors take a very methodical and logical approach to tasks and are more concerned with the process than they are with the outcome. These individuals are deliberate in their approach, focusing on planning, systemizing, and orchestrating plans in a sequential manner. They will typically make lists to help them track their progress during the day or week. They enjoy completing each task and checking or crossing off each item as it is completed. If this is your style, you understand this. They enjoy working alone and need little assistance from others to complete their tasks.

Let's take a closer look at the characteristics of the processor. They are described as individuals who are more subdued and patient. They truly enjoy gathering data and working alone on specific projects. They tend to gear themselves toward operations because they are very precise, and operations reflect more of a systematic process. They have extremely high standards and can become frustrated with those who do not reflect these standards. They do not enjoy conflict but not for the same reason as the politician or the peacemaker. Their reason is because, in their minds, conflict does not need to exist because if they have worked on a project, it is correct and the outcome is accurate. They are not excited about change because, in their minds, change usually means a new set of procedures and structures they would have to learn to have a sense of consistency and accuracy. Finally, they are not great team players. It is not that they don't enjoy people or enjoy socializing but mainly because they find that they are able to accomplish outcomes on their own in a more accurate manner than with a group.

As I stated to you, processors can be the most misunderstood individuals because of how they are perceived by others. When you ask processors what they think, they will say that they feel that they are team players, although others might not see them in the same light.

Are you starting to recognize the people you work with who have this personality style? Mostly likely this personality style gravitates towards those types of roles that involve more data gathering and data management, such as quality assurance and performance improvement initiatives.

This personality is special to me because my wife, who is a staff nurse in a postsurgical setting, is a processor, and she has provided me with excellent examples of how this style works. If you are looking to have your staff assume responsibility for creating an excellent caregiving atmosphere, processors are wonderful to have. They are committed to excellence. They focus on how things are operationalized in a unit or program and are usually vocal about what works and what doesn't work. They will point out your areas of deficiency and identify operations that are lacking. However, because they are very accurate and committed to excellence, they are seen by others as "know-it-alls." In addition, they are not as committed to working together as a team and can be seen as cold and aloof. They are highly valuable people to have in your work setting, and all efforts must be made to identify how to retain and develop these health care workers. They will bring you excellence.

Here is what staff say about peers with a processor style.

- "I don't understand them."
- "They always want to do it their way."
- "They are always dependable."

Staff who are processors are

1. consistent and dependable: you can trust them,
2. rigid in process; they follow the policies,
3. misunderstood because they prefer to work alone.

When it comes to being fair and consistent, these are the people for the job. Processing supervisors pride themselves on their accuracy and consistency with all employees. Unlike the peacemaker and the politician, the processor will assure that all policies and procedures and employee expectations are held consistent for each staff member. This is seen as a very positive and supportive endeavor by all employees.

Initially, they may come across as harsh and difficult, but through time and understanding, the style can be viewed by staff as competent and dependable.

Getting to that point can be the most difficult challenge for processing supervisors. Because of their need to work alone, it is hard to support a shared governance or teamwork decision model. They have a tendency to grow quickly frustrated with the lack of movement or decision making by a team or the inability of that team to think in the same manner they do, (much like pointers). What this can lead to is a lack of trust and support from the employees.

This is what staff say about supervisors with the processor style.

- "I love working for her. I understand what is expected of me."
- "I like her because she doesn't play favorites; she is fair with everyone."
- "Can she ever be flexible? She is so rigid, and she is not capable of just sitting down to talk."

Supervisors who are processors

1. are fair and consistent with all staff,
2. focus on all policies and procedures,
3. can be rigid as a result of being consistent.

Based on your evaluation scores and the descriptions, you now know your own 4-P Personality Style. Most people have one dominant style. Dominant styles are very telling. Not only is it your most natural style from which to operate, you also tend to gravitate toward your dominant style when you are stressed or overextended.

Have you clearly identified your style? Does it make sense to you? Have you identified your peers' and supervisors' styles? Does it answer questions you have had about their behavior? It should. At this point, you should have a different understanding of the people with whom you work. I hope you do.

Identifying the Personality Styles of Others

We spent a great deal of time talking about your personality style, what it looks like, and how it plays out under periods of extreme stress, but now that you understand these four personality styles, I want you to be able to identify other's personality styles. Why is that important to you? As we move into the upcoming truths about managing difficult personalities and developing dynamic teams, it is imperative that you are able to recognize these styles so you can clearly and effectively communicate your ideas.

In review of the 4-P personality styles, we know the following.

1. You have to understand your own personality style and the characteristics that surround that personality style.
2. You can understand that others do not share your way of thinking or processing information, even though they may have the same goals as you do in the workplace setting.
3. For you to be successful, you want to be able to quickly identify the personality styles of other people with whom you interact.

This may seem daunting, but actually it is not, especially during periods of stress. During periods of stress, people demonstrate their dominant personality style. Again, I want to take this time to reiterate. Even though from your test you may have had multiple or very close personality styles, according to your score, you will gravitate towards a dominant personality style during those periods and times of stress. Review your characteristics grid. During periods of stress, pointers direct, processors isolate and work, peacemakers take care of others, and politicians socialize.

So how do we do this? An easy solution is asking open-ended questions to identify how somebody responds. For example, when I am interacting with a patient or family that I have not met before, I will ask the simple question "How can I help you?" or "What do you need?" The four personality styles will respond differently.

The Pointer:
Question: "What do you need?"
Answer: "I'll tell you what I need . . ."

The pointer's response will be very direct and focused on outcomes, and they need it yesterday.

The Processor:
Question: "What do you need?"
Answer: "I brought a list with me of the questions that I have, and I would like you to answer them for me."

If they do have a list with them, it will be in sequential processing order, such as a, b, c or 1, 2, 3.

The Peacemaker:
Question: "What do you need?"
Answer: "Nothing, I am fine. Is there anything I can do for you?"

This may sound silly, but peacemakers are the easiest patients and families to interact with.

The Politician:
Question: "What do you need?"
Answer: "I am not sure. I don't really understand what's occurring. Can we talk about it?"

The politician will want to sit down and have a discussion regarding what is occurring. It is usually nonspecific, and they much prefer doing this over a cup of coffee.

As difficult as it may appear to try to analyze different individuals, you are really just evaluating their communication style. During times of hospitalization or in the service care arena, we find that, more likely than not, individuals are at a higher stress level, thus demonstrating more openly their specific personality style. Remember why you are doing this. It is not in order to control them but so that you can communicate more effectively, put them in a place of control, and reduce their stress. It is helpful to observe patterns of behavior over time, rather than make an assessment from one isolated incident. Although this is not always possible, such as in when you step into a conflict without knowing the parties involved, it will generally help you make a more accurate assessment.

Once you know someone else's style, you can present information in a way they can actually hear it. Not only will it make your life easier, it will appeal to the other person as well. Even if they do not realize what you are doing, they will feel respected and cared for, which is always helpful when you are working in stressful conditions.

When you do not know each other's styles, miscommunication is easy, often resulting in unintended conflict. As you continue to miscommunicate, the conflict will escalate.

Here is an example of how not being aware of personality styles can result in detrimental conflict and how using personality styles information helped transform the conflict into a collaborative effort.

I was called in to consult for a hospital in the Midwest. The hospital was attempting to open an additional med/surge wing and wanted some assistance completing this task. When I arrived, I met the nurse manager first. She was pleasant and reviewed the overall plan, including scheduled staff training to deal with the transition to a new unit. She also told me that another matter had arisen that needed my immediate attention. I asked her to explain.

She instructed me to walk on the unit and view the nurse's station and said that would better explain the situation. As I left her office and walked to the nurse's station, I noticed something strange in the middle of the desk. On the desk was bright pink tape laid out in a complete square about 12 inches by 12 inches. The area around this square was neatly kept, and the chair at this station was pushed against the desk in an orderly way. This was puzzling because the rest of the nurse's station had chairs pulled out, and some charts and a great deal of paperwork in disarray covered the area. The area with the tape, however, was pristine, almost as if no one dare disturb this area of the desk.

I returned to the manager to review what I had seen. As I explained, I watched as the nurse manager's face became tense and she began to lean forward. I asked her if she could provide me with an explanation. She stated, "About two and a half months ago, I noticed our staff having conflict. They always had been a close group, celebrating birthdays at work, having holiday parties, and even socializing outside the hospital, but that changed, and much of this has to do with our unit clerk, Becky."

A dependable worker, it appeared that Becky had divided the unit and severely affected the morale and patient care. I asked how one person could do this and, if she did, why? The manager didn't know. Numerous meetings to address Becky's behavior resulted in no change. The manager issued verbal warnings and then written warnings, all to no avail. But what about the tape on the desk?

The manager told me it was Becky's latest move. The previous week Becky had been counseled about failing to file specific papers. Becky told the manager that the desk was such a mess she could not find these papers, and they became lost. She stated she would make sure this did not happen again. The next day Becky had marked her area and stated that any work needing to be done had to be put inside the box. If the work were not placed in the box, she would not be held accountable. The manager could not believe what she was hearing.

I asked the manager again how things had gotten so bad. She just shook her head and could not answer me. I asked her, "So what do you want from me?" She replied, "I need you to work with her and pull the staff together."

Later that afternoon, I approached Becky and introduced myself. Without leaving her chair, she looked up at me and stated, "I know why you're here, and I want nothing to do with you." Startled but not put off, I asked again to speak with her, this time adding a little laughter to the situation. "If you don't see me, I will have to go home, and it's a long drive at night to Cincinnati." With a blank stare, she said, "Goodbye." Dejected, I decided to wait until the next morning. When she saw me coming toward the nurse's station, she looked away. I asked her for just 15 minutes of her time. I'm not sure why, and I don't think she knew either, but she agreed to meet with me.

From the moment she began speaking, it was clear that Becky needed to be in control of the conversation. It did not take long for me to tell she was a pointer, and I made sure I let her take control of the conversation. As a result, I discovered she did not mind that the 15 minutes quickly extended to 30 minutes and then to an hour. She began feeling comfortable with me because she never felt out of control. Then I used the phrase that all pointers love to hear: "I need your help." I asked her if she could help me do my job of bringing the unit back together. She told me she was not sure how to do that but that she did have some ideas.

Becky began by telling me what everyone else had done to break this unit apart. I asked her when all this began. Without hesitation, she told me of a day 2½ months before, that was clear in her mind. She proudly explained that she had been the staff member with the longest employment and saw herself as the one who coordinated and directed all the activities for the staff outside of the hospital. One day as she was walking to the break room where a report was given, she heard two nurses planning the surprise party for another co-worker. (Traditionally, this had been her role). As she entered the room, the two nurses became startled and left the room.

Two days later, an invitation came to the staff regarding the surprise party from the two nurses. Immediately, Becky was approached by other staff asking if she knew about this. Embarrassed and angry, Becky began to shut down and focus her energy on the nurses who planned the party. She told me, "Who did they think they are? This is what I do. I'm the one who organizes these things."

After another hour, she had told me the whole story. She looked relieved that she was able to talk about this on her terms (pointer) but also sad about her present situation with the staff and the unit. Soon after, she became tearful and just wanted everything to be the same as it was.

The next day, I met with Becky and the two nurses. It was not easy to get them in the same room together. For the last 2 months, the anger between Becky and the nurses had grown. Lines were drawn among the staff, with everyone choosing sides (except the peacemaker who just wanted everyone to stop fighting).

It was clear that within the first 10 minutes, that Joan (one of the nurses) was a pointer as well. Her sidekick, Martha, was a peacemaker, following Joan's lead. Martha only spoke when Joan looked at her, and she never interrupted. I explained that I was going to review what I knew and then give everyone a chance to clarify. Knowing the personality styles I was dealing with, I made sure to just present the facts and make my point quickly; too much detail and I would lose their interest.

After meeting for 30 minutes, both sides were able to agree on the facts. At this point, I introduced the 4-P Personality Styles model. They were eager to hear more. It was as if a boulder had been lifted from all of their shoulders. They got it! Becky and Joan understood they both needed to be in control and that's just who they are. After that, we began to outline how they could co-exist on the unit. For the next 3 days, Becky, Joan, Martha, and I met with all the staff, processing the last 5 weeks and introducing the personality styles. The group had advanced to the point that they could laugh at each other's style with acceptance and without making judgments. Understanding these personality styles and letting people be in control was the key for the entire staff to stop arguing and begin healing.

What was quickly escalating into job frustration, burnout, and potentially a negative effect on patient care was easily addressed through the 4-P Personality Styles. By addressing this first element of the Circle of Control, you can easily shift the overall experience of the caregiver.

Specific Self-Worth

When we speak of self-worth, a general glaze comes over many people's eyes. Because the term has been used over and over again, it now has little meaning to most people. They nod in understanding, without actually thinking about what self-esteem really means.

Have you looked on the Internet lately? Type "self-worth" into a search engine, and you will find numerous Websites telling you how to improve yours. They identify signs of low self-esteem and what healthy self-esteem is. With so many people providing so many different interpretations, how can anyone understand exactly how this fits into your life and your Circle of Control?

When I speak about specific self-worth, I am less interested in a list that you feel describes who you are than I am in an identification of what you perceive your inner self to be, and, more specifically, what is most important to you. Others would call this really

> **Specific self-worth is a sequential list of how you perceive yourself— what is <u>most</u> important to you?**

knowing who you are or really having a good sense of yourself. According to Belitz and Lungstrom, authors of *Power of Flow: Practical Ways To Transform Your Life With Meaningful Coincidence*, your level of self-worth is the difference between who you think you ought to be or want to be and who you judge yourself to be. This is a very important statement because as we look at specific self-worth, I am asking you to identify who you think you want to be and what the priorities of those characteristics are. More importantly, if the time that you spend throughout the day does not support your priority list, your level of self-esteem will be less.

Doesn't this make sense? When we talk about your Circle of Control and living life consciously, understanding who you are as it relates to what your day-to-day efforts are is very powerful. The sequential order of what you hold dear to yourself has to be supported by your day-to-day actions, and the only way this can occur is for you to be conscious of exactly what those priorities are in your life.

For example, if the priorities in life that define you are mother-hood, career, and friendship (in that order), your daily actions would then have to support this order. Does the amount of time you spend each day support being a mother first, then your career? If it doesn't, for whatever reason, you will actually experience internal conflict and a diminished sense of self-worth. You are not in sync.

I met with a very successful career woman, Susan, who graduated from a prestigious university and became an accomplished lawyer. Susan moved on to the television industry where she began to learn producing and directing. After 10 years in this field, she took her talents to a national news magazine where she dedicated her days to being the best at her craft. In a short period, her efforts paid off, and she went on to a successful career, winning four Emmy awards. Still feeling unfulfilled, she moved her energies in another direc-tion, deciding to move from behind the camera to in front as a TV sports announcer. She again took the same rigorous work ethic to achieve her goals. Again, she was successful. She received awards and praise from others, but still Susan did not feel fulfilled. I met Susan at this point in her career. In my meetings with her, it was quite clear that she continued to search for a sense of happiness through a variety of different career changes. As we sat down to identify her Circle of Control and specific self-worth characteristics, it became evident that her career goals were not her initial priority.

She told me that she wanted most of all to become a mother and had had several failed relationships. Susan was very sensitive about this issue. She became very defensive when others discussed this, especially family. To deal with this disappointment, she decided to pour her energies into her career. However, this didn't work. Susan found no fulfillment or satisfaction no matter how successful she became in her career. Her most important goal was to become a mother, yet all of her daily actions were spent on another activity.

After defining her specific self-worth characteristics, Susan was able to understand why she continued to feel bad about herself. She stated that it continued to feel as if she could not quench her thirst no matter what she did. She understood why she reacted neg-atively when individuals talked about family to her. She understood why she became defensive and managed that anger through avoid-ance and throwing herself into her career. Once Susan began this process of being conscious about herself and identifying her Circle of Control, she began to feel a sense of peace. She told me for the first time in her life she did not feel like she had to prove anything.

Her anxiety left her. Today Susan is married, has a child, and balances her priorities.

This is just an example of understanding the importance of identifying your specific self-worth, knowing your priorities, and ensuring your daily actions support them. By addressing your self-worth, you can extend your Circle of Control. What does your list look like?

Below is the specific self-worth worksheet for you to complete. The first column is your list, and the second column is actual evidence (time spent) that supports your ratings. Please take your time and think about each item. Be honest and accurate about how much time you actually spend on each characteristic.

For the evidence section, I want you to identify the number of hours each day you spend on each characteristics. Assuming you sleep 7–9 hours each night, you have up to 15–17 hours each day to account for. For example, Susan identified being a supportive, loving wife and mother as her #1 characteristics. However, time spent each day was less than 2 hours. "Successful employer/ professional" was second on her list but time spent each exceeded 10 hours per day. You can see the internal conflict.

External Support Systems

Identifying your personality style and knowing your most important specific self-worth characteristics are the most important aspects of

SPECIFIC SELF-WORTH WORKSHEET

PRIORITY LIST	EVIDENCE
1.	
2.	
3.	
4.	
5.	

your Circle of Control. I have found, however, that without having the ability to share these dynamics with others in your life, you are unable to validate and reevaluate the process of growth for yourself. It makes applying and sustaining your changes virtually impossible. Sharing this journey with those around you helps to validate it for you, reinforcing your commitment to developing your Circle of Control.

Quite simply, you need to identify the support systems in your life both at work and at home. You need to share the dynamics of your personality style and your specific self-worth characteristics with them. Once they have this information and understand you better, you can ask them to help support you through this process. These key support people also aid you when life is difficult and you need their reassurance to stay on your path.

Who are these individuals? You might call them your brother, parent, best friend, or coworker, those you feel close enough to to share your Circle of Control. Some nurses I have spoken with talk to me about long-distance friendships they continue to maintain because they have a special bond that even distance does not break. This is what I am speaking of when I talk about external support systems. For most of you, it will be just one to three people in your life. Whatever the number is, you need to share with these people your Circle of Control and request that they provide feedback to you when you begin to veer from your Circle of Control, acting in ways that do not support it.

Becoming conscious of your circle is your first goal. You must bring to light the three variables of your Circle of Control and claim responsibility for their impact on your environment. Then by applying these principles, you can determine how your life will be different. In the case of Becky, she was able to identify the source of her anger and ways to meet her needs, reconnect with her coworkers, and stop the pain. For Susan, it was becoming conscious of her true priorities and ensuring that her daily actions supported these. Susan told me that once she made this list and her actions become conscious and purposeful, her stress and anger lifted.

Consciously living with your Circle of Control can be a difficult task. It is also rewarding. With your support systems around you, an appreciation of your specific self-worth, and a keen understanding of personality style, you can take exquisite care of the caregiver—yourself. As you couple this understanding with the Success Steps in Truth #3, you will experience a new sense of relief, excitement, and hope.

ACHIEVING SUCCESS WITH EVERY CONVERSATION

The Success Steps Model

We have two ears and one tongue so that we would listen more and talk less.

—Diogenes

Congratulations! You have steered your way through the first two truths. You have a better understanding of who you are and your own Circle of Control. By now, you have a different understanding of yourself. You also see things in a different light. As a result of understanding the 4-P Personality Styles, you not only understand yourself but those around you. You are able to view each relationship in your life from a different perspective. In addition to this, you also see your family and friends differently. Some of you may have a sense of peace and contentment about yourself because you understand why you have reacted to others the way you have. Others have described to me that they feel a door has opened up for them. As in Susan's story, for the first time, they feel a sense of peace and contentment. I hope you are experiencing this at this time as well. As we move forward to the third truth, you are going to learn additional techniques that, coupled with your Circle of Control, will help you successfully manage each of your interactions with others.

Success Steps

I created the Success Steps model to provide you with a guide for managing your interactions with others for the purpose of achieving your desired outcome or, minimally, just understanding the outcome that has resulted. As with the 4-P Personality Styles, I have developed these steps with the assistance of many other colleagues along the way. During my 20 years in the health care and service industries, I became intrigued with the idea of how to get people to do what I wanted them to do. With so many people reacting in different ways to my requests, I wanted to understand how to best meet their needs and guide my interactions to develop a positive outcome. Let me tell you, there is a lot of trial and error in developing this, but it works. The Success Steps model has been founded and tested in principle and has provided me as well as hundreds of other health care personnel with a tool to improve their experiences at work and home.

> **The Success Steps provide you with a guide for managing your interactions to achieve your outcomes.**

The beauty of the Success Steps model is that it is simple. I created it after being in several situations in which I did not know how to respond or what to say. How many times have you been given different theories and tools that are too complicated to remember? If the tool is not simple and easy enough to use immediately, you will not use it. It is very unlikely that you will refer to a manual while you are interacting with someone else; by the time you do, it is much too late, and your window of opportunity has passed.

As you progress through each step, learn each of the elements and consider how you could use them in specific situations in your own life. Not only will this help you understand the model, it will help you remember the principles the next time you are in the heat of the moment, when you really need it.

Each of the Success Steps has its own unique principles and is designed to work in a sequential manner, providing a path for managing each interaction you have, and moving you toward achieving your true outcomes. Because the steps are sequential, you must

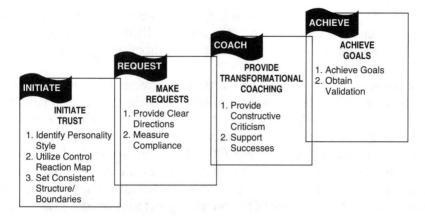

The Success Steps Model to Emotional Connection

proceed through them *in order* with each person with whom you interact. Failure to do so will result in even greater frustration for you and for the other person.

Knowing why people react the way they do, and having the ability to understand exactly what to say next in a conversation or a difficult situation, provides you with a sense of confidence and control over your day. The Success Steps model does exactly that. It will increase your sense of self and your sense of control by achieving your goals despite the changes occurring in your external world. As with any tool, if used improperly, it becomes ineffective at best and detrimental at worst. It is important to understand the rules of using this tool.

The situation can change moment to moment, and this can be frustrating. With this tool, however, you can know immediately what is happening and adjust your strategy accordingly. Again, you are determining which of your actions will give you the desired reaction. Based on verbal and nonverbal responses, you will know exactly on which step someone is located. Understanding why people react the way they do and being able to anticipate their next reaction is powerful. This is what the Success Steps model does. Can you imagine how much easier your work—and life—will be when you can apply this tool? I promise you will feel a new sense of empowerment as a result of this model.

Before we begin to evaluate the four steps in the Success Steps model, you must understand the core fundamental rules. These rules will provide you with a greater understanding of the Success Steps operational procedures.

Rule #1: Before you can use the Success Steps model, you must have successfully completed the first two truth steps. This means you have to have a conscious understanding of your reality and your Circle of Control.

Rule #2: The goal of the Success Steps model is to better understand how to meet the needs of the individual you are speaking with, not control him or her. If you are attempting to control somebody, you will fail. This model is based on respect for and better understanding of those with whom you are speaking.

Rule #3: Every time you interact with people, they are trying to convey a message. For some, it can be a simple welcoming; for others, it can be an attempt to convince you to follow their direction. In the range of interactions, the approach stays the same. The Success Steps model will help you achieve your goals.

Rule #4: During each interaction, all participants will be located on one of the four steps. Based on the individual, you can determine your next interventions to move the individual through each step of the model. The end goal is to reach Step Four, Achieve Goals.

Rule #5: The most important element of this model is that you must successfully achieve each step in a sequential manner. If you attempt to skip a step, you will discover individuals remaining on Step One, Initiate Trust.

Rule #6: At any given moment, individuals can move up or down on the Success Steps model. Relationships can be fragile. Something someone says or does can erode confidence in an individual, resulting in "falling down the stairs" to Step One. Let's begin with Step One, Initiate Trust.

Step One: Initiate Trust

How many books have you read that talk about developing trust? It almost seems as if it is an overused phrase that gets little attention. Throughout my career it has been the most crucial step in the model. In fact, I have identified that 60% of my time is spent on this step. Moreover, as I have consulted with several health care organizations, I have noticed that many of them continue to operate on step one. Many have done this for so long, it is normal to them, and they do not know what it is like to move beyond this. As we move into the upcoming truths, we will talk about using this model both for managing difficult personalities and creating a dynamic team.

> **60% of your time will be spent on Step One of the Success Steps model.**

Therefore, when you talk about trust, it can appear to be a very general term. However, I am here to tell you that it is not. It has several components. It can be broken down into measurable aspects. As we progress, we will evaluate these different aspects of trust.

In an article, from the *Harvard Business Review* (March 2004) Sajnicole A. Joni, author of *The Geography of Trust*, supported the importance of trust in an organization yet pondered how little scrutiny it receives. She further breaks trust into two specific areas, one called personal trust and the other structural trust. She goes on to say that personal trust is usually based on faith and a person's integrity. It's probably the most fundamental and widely understood trust. Continuing, she says that "Higher personal trust exists when we answer 'yes' to the following questions: Is this person ethical? Will he or she make good on his word? Is he or she well intentioned? Will he or she handle confidential information with care and discretion? Will he or she be straightforward about what he or she does not know?"

Structural trust refers more to how roles and ambition affect the insight and information provided to both managers and leaders. Basically, it's the politics of an organization and how that relates to individual staff trust. I support Ms. Joni's description of both kinds of trust, and I do find that many nationally known authors discuss trust on this level. Where I take exception to this is the lack of measurement of what trust is and how you know you have obtained it.

What I am saying is that staff need to understand how you obtain and maintain trust during each interaction. During each interaction, you will be given an opportunity to gain or lose trust. I know that some of you may be thinking that it's the choice of others whether or not they choose to give their trust. However, these tools will place you in a much better position to earn it. Each time you initiate a conversation, whether it is with someone you have met for the first time or a peer that you work with daily, you will have the opportunity to create trust with that individual. Haven't you ever wondered why some people like you and others do not? Why you have trusted some and others you have not? Or, why some people interpret your interactions differently than do other people? There are a great many reasons of why this occurs. For the majority of you it is because trust has not been developed. Remember, it does not just happen. When we reviewed personality styles, we were able to identify why you relate better to styles that reflect your own. As we begin to evaluate the different aspects of trust, you will have to believe that you will be given all the tools you need to make this happen. Let's begin by evaluating the six guidelines to gaining trust.

Guideline #1: All of us want to be in control. If at any time you find yourself in an interaction with others and you attempt to control them, you will have failed.

Guideline #2: All individuals in an interaction want to feel in control and manage the conversation. Based on their personality styles, they identify control in different ways.

Guideline #3: The perception of being in or out of control can directly affect your sense of self or identity. What I am saying is when you feel in control, you feel better about yourself. The reverse is also true. When you feel out of control, you become defensive and react accordingly.

Guideline #4: There is a predictable pattern among those individuals who feel out of control. When control is taken away from individuals and they do feel out of control, they will "act out." (A definition of what acting out is will be provided later). They will also socialize negatively with their peers and supervisors.

Guideline #5: When people perceive themselves to be in control, they do not feel threatened or become defensive and thus do not need to regain control. When you feel that you are in control, your reaction is to return control to others and socialize positively.

Guideline #6: How you interact with others will directly affect their perception and their feelings of being in or out of control. This process is called the Control Reaction Map. It is a guideline for you to understand and to measure specifically if an individual is feeling in or out of control.

Step One of the Success Steps model consists of three components. Each of these will be reviewed in detail.

1. Determining the 4-P Personality Style
2. Successfully navigating the Control Reaction Map
3. Setting appropriate boundaries and structure

To achieve trust you must accomplish each component. We have already reviewed the 4-P Personality Styles in truth #2. Let's evaluate the last two components.

The Control Reaction Map

The Control Reaction Map was designed as a practical guide for all your interactions. It will provide for you a road map to achieving trust. During your interactions with others, each area is being evaluated (consciously or unconsciously) at the same time. Often we are just not aware of these areas, except for the outcome of feeling in or out of control. By being aware of this map you can make adjustments in your interaction to reach the outcome you desire.

Take your time and review each aspect of the Control Reaction Map. There are five different aspects. We have discussed in detail the Circle of Control in the second truth. Understanding your personality style and those around you is essential for the initial step.

The goal of the Control Reaction Map is to move individuals to the fourth aspect (outcome) and to have a sense of feeling in control. If you refer to the fourth aspect of the Control Reaction Map (outcomes), you can see that all of us have two choices—the choice of feeling in or out of control. The results of these choices are dramatically different. How you manage the first three aspects of this map will contribute significantly to the feeling of being in or out of control. When an individual feels in control, you have gained trust and are successful with Step One of the Success Steps model.

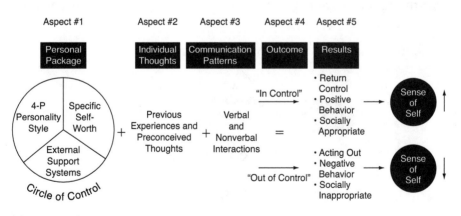

The Control Reaction Map

> **The Control Reaction Map was designed as a practical guide to achieving trust.**

Let's look at each of these aspects.

Aspects of the Control Reaction Map

Personal Package
In the second truth, we reviewed extensively your Circle of Control. We also established your individual 4-P Personality Style and how to determine others' styles. We spent time on what questions you can ask that will assist you in this process. As for determining others' specific self-worth and external support systems, this can be more complicated, mainly because if an individual has not determined this themselves, it can be difficult for you to do it. What you can do is be aware of others' defenses or sensitive issues. During your interaction with peers or patients, be aware of topics or areas that cause individuals to turn away from you or minimize your interaction. You do not have to know the issue; just understand they are struggling with it.

Individual Thoughts
All of us have preconceived thoughts and previous experiences. Some are great, some are not so great. Each of these experiences and thoughts will affect our interactions with others. Most of your

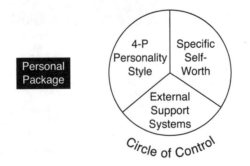

Personal Package

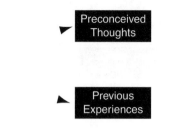

Individual Thoughts

patients have had past experiences with nurses and hospital personnel. These experiences will affect how they interact with you. They may be guarded, anticipating a poor interaction. This is true for you as well as your peers.

Why is that important? You can see that you begin to progress towards the track of feeling out of control. If you are to gain trust with an individual, you have to be aware of these preconceived thoughts and these previous experiences.

So what do you do about this? If there has been a misunderstanding or if there has been a negative experience with an individual, you may have to address this experience. In some cases, it is enough to just acknowledge that this is a new situation and the results from past experiences do not have to be the same. Remember what we discussed earlier. If you enter into a power struggle, you will not move any closer to achieving trust in Step One of the Success Steps model. I repeat this because I have witnessed it. In these situations, there is such a need to be right that trust is never gained.

Communication Patterns
Understanding how an individual is responding (or reacting) to your interaction is the most important aspect of the Control Reaction Map. This is because you can visually see whether someone is moving closer toward feeling in or out of control. This includes verbal and nonverbal interactions. Think about this. When you are interacting with somebody who does not trust you, what does that sound like? Most likely, it's responses that are

- short answers
- sarcastic rebuttals
- nonspecific answers

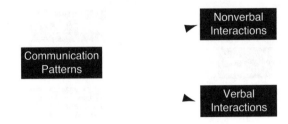

Communication Patterns

And what would the nonverbal responses look like for the individual who doesn't trust you?

- very closed posture, possibly arms folded
- poor eye contact
- a turned-away posture/different height posture (standing over someone)

It is very important that you be conscious of the verbal and nonverbal responses of the individual with whom you are speaking. As you implement the first three aspects of the Control Reaction Map, you can begin to understand the interconnectedness of each aspect. You want to determine the personality style with which you are dealing, and you want to acknowledge if there have been any negative past experiences.

In a book by Jo-Ellan Dimitrius, *How to Understand People and Predict Their Behavior Anytime, Anyplace,* she focuses on reading verbal and nonverbal patterns in others to determine what they want. She states, "You have to be aware that there can be hidden meanings in communication with others." She further states, "I've seen many well-meaning and candid witnesses initially appear evasive, only to demonstrate later that they were trying their best to respond. You have to really listen to what others are and are not saying."

Results

Let's look at the last aspect of the Control Reaction Map, which is the results of each outcome. With each outcome, individuals demonstrate two very different responses. When people feel in control, they will demonstrate certain behaviors. These behaviors are positive and demonstrate that you have gained their trust. This is your goal for this first step. Let's identify what this looks like.

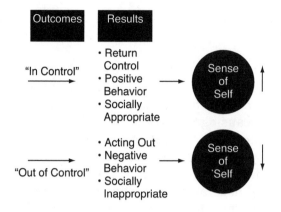

Outcomes and Results

- The individual returns control to you through compliments, support, etc.
- Positive behavior is demonstrated. The person is optimistic and helpful, often described as a "team" player.
- Socially appropriate phrases such as "please" and "thank you" are used.

For those who are feeling out of control in an interaction with you, the results will be vastly different. Demonstration of these behaviors will inform you that you have not gained trust and that you need to reevaluate your map and plan another interaction. Let's evaluate these behaviors. First, those feeling out of control may exhibit acting-out behaviors. We talked about this in the form of socially inappropriate behavior and responses. These people may yell, avoid you, or refuse to speak with you.

In the end, those who perceive themselves to be out of control create a decreased sense of self, and those who perceive themselves to be in control create an increased sense of self. When you begin to look at experiences in your life, you can see how this occurs. Self-esteem is enhanced when you achieve. Feeling out of control does not produce a sense of accomplishment. It is just the opposite.

Employees who feel they have lost control at work will find ways to take control. You have probably seen this in your own workplace. Examples of these acting-out behaviors are sick calls, refusing to work with certain individuals, unrealistic demands on peers and supervisors, and the ultimate in acting-out behavior, quitting. Patients perceiving themselves to be out of control may act in similar ways. They may refuse to follow your directions, become noncompliant or argumentative.

These acting-out behaviors are an attempt to regain control. These behaviors affect everyone. As we discussed, it produces a lowered sense of self, further affecting the situation. It can be a negative cycle, causing everyone around to be defensive for the purpose of protecting themselves. Can you understand why they act the way they do? It may not change the situation, but it changes your understanding and, ultimately, your perception.

The most popular way of protecting one's sense of self is avoidance. Most of us tend to avoid those we do not like. Most of you have practiced this technique.

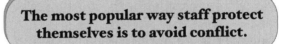

The most popular way staff protect themselves is to avoid conflict.

Doesn't this make sense? You do not want to risk feeling worse about yourself, so you remove yourself from the situation. However, there are others who respond to a loss of self in a different manner. They respond by attempting to decrease the other person's sense of self by attempting to hurt their feelings. They talk about others, ostracize them, and even confront them in a negative manner. It is not pretty. They want everyone to be as miserable as they are. Misery loves company.

Until individuals develop a sense of trust, they will continue this cycle of feeling out of control. They will continue to act out, demonstrate negative behavior, and socialize inappropriately. For those of you caught in this cycle, you do not have to continue experiencing this. Decide you want to create a new experience and begin implementing these truths.

What we do not realize is that we believe we can avoid individuals that we don't like, this can be peers, patients, or families. The reality is we can't. We will interact with them at some point, and as a result of avoiding them, both parties interact in a negative manner through attention seeking. The patients we ignore receive our attention by identifying problems with care, frequent call lights, and using their family to complain. With our peers and supervisors that we don't like, we interact in a negative manner. The interaction usually takes place under duress. It may be an argument, sarcasm, or it may be the use of jokes. Why do we do this? Again we do not feel comfortable and safe, and this is an attempt to get our needs met. You have to understand this.

Let's go back to the story of Becky from the second truth. When I first introduced myself to her, Becky was feeling out of control because she assumed I was there to "deal" with her behavior (preconceived thoughts). This made her defensive. She also didn't know me and had no reason to trust me, particularly given the circumstances she had been dealing with already. She is a great example of how hard it can be to develop trust with certain individuals. There may be numerous reasons why someone doesn't trust you that you may never be able to identify. That is OK, as long as you recognize *how* they are expressing themselves and continue to work to help them feel in control.

In Becky's case, I chose to let her have that control each time I approached her. I did not push or become frustrated. I recognized her discomfort at my being there to meet with her. Her communication patterns were negative, and her personality style was controlling. I continued to adjust my approach to achieve the desired outcome of having Becky feel in control. Becky was defensive and acting out, so I chose to continue to offer my assistance and let her be in control until her defenses lowered. How did I know this? Remember, I could tell she was feeling in control because she started to return control to me and interact more positively than when we first began speaking.

If I had become impatient or frustrated, Becky would have continued to rebel and act out. Her interaction with me would have continued to be hostile. By letting her direct the conversation, I placed her in a position of control. This occurred because I agreed to her rules of how we were going to interact and continually asked her opinion of the entire situation. Not only did this put her in a place of control, it resulted in her feeling better about herself, and thus we began to develop a socialization pattern of respect. I had accomplished the first step with Becky, and I was ready to move on to Step Two of the Success Steps model (Request).

Structure and Boundaries

Great job! You have successfully completed the first two components of Step One of the Success Steps model (Identifying the 4-P

Personality Style and Control Reaction Map). Let's look at the third component—setting structure and boundaries.

Setting boundaries and structure is an integral part of helping people perceive they are in control, and during my seminars, it is one of the things I am most asked about. They want to understand what it means. The best way to answer this is that consistent structure and boundaries provide individuals with a sense of safety and security. Let me elaborate on this point.

According to Jeri Minchington, author of *Maximum Self-Esteem: The Handbook for Reclaiming your Sense of Self-Worth*, a lack of structure and a lack of boundaries in in your life can lead to a decrease in a sense of self. In the long run, this decreased sense of self will lead you to consistently remain on Step One, always feeling out of control. By providing a sense of structure (expectations) in your daily routine, others know how to interact with you and what to expect during these interactions. Through boundaries and structure, you can measure if you have achieved. It is through achievement that you enhance your self-worth. You are more likely to perceive you are in control if you are able to understand what is expected of you, decreasing your defensiveness.

Doesn't this make sense? This is why we create rules and guidelines—not to control others, but to put them in a place to succeed.

Achievement is more readily attained if clear expectations are stated. In addition, you are more likely to achieve in a setting where boundaries and structure are constant. As we talk further in truth five, developing a dynamic team, we will review the role of specific structures and boundaries that put people in a place to succeed and allow them to more readily feel in control, thus gaining trust.

Step Two: Make Requests

You must obtain someone's trust in order to be successful in the next step, Make Requests. Without trust they will not follow your requests, leaving everyone frustrated. You want people to do what you have asked of them, not because of a need to be important, but because it's important to the functioning and welfare of the team and patients. You want your patients to follow your instructions. Their health depends on it. You also attempt to convince your colleagues and influence your managers and supervisors to share your perspective on issues. You know that without establishing trust, individuals will not follow your direction. (Fear might work, but only for a while).

Asking people to do things is what you do as a nurse and a health care professional. You position yourself to win the trust of patients and families so they will follow your instructions. Some would say, "I'll do what you want because I respect you." What they are really saying is, "You were able to articulate yourself in a way that made me trust you, and now I will follow your directions." Measuring the compliance of a request will be very important when determining if you can move on to the next of the Success Steps.

The largest mistake that people make in interactions is assuming that because a request was not carried out, it means the individual does not trust you. This is not always the case. It may be because the individual did not understand exactly what you wanted or did not have the proper tools to complete the task. This occurs frequently in health care organizations. The assumption is made that staff who do not follow management direction do not want to comply with the request. They are described as having a poor attitude. In most situations, the reason for not following a direction is not understanding what was requested or not having the proper systems in place to complete the task. The effort was there, the attitude was there, the energy was there, but staff did not have the tools to be able to finish or complete the desired request. Chances are they probably were not aware of it.

It is important to understand this difference. Blaming staff or patients for not completing a task when they did not have the correct tools will only return you to Step One and place a roadblock to regaining trust.

So what do you do if someone does not comply with your request once you have determined that they clearly understood what was asked of them? You return to Step One to determine why there is a lack of trust. With Becky, after I made my initial request and she quickly thwarted my efforts to meet with her, I did not continue to pursue that request. I stopped. I stepped back. I gave her time, which helped her feel in control by allowing her to set the tone. Then my request to meet with her was granted. In fact, she quickly extended her initial time parameters.

However, this is not the path Becky's manager chose. The manager moved quickly past Step One and into Step Two. This is a common management mistake. (We will cover this at greater length in the seventh truth.) The manager told me that she brought Becky in on three separate occasions. The first time she asked her what was wrong. Becky responded, "Nothing." She attempted again, with Becky giving the same response. She then did what a majority of people do when they experience feeling out of control; she moved on to Step Two and began making requests without first building trust. She did this by giving her a verbal then a written warning. It's not difficult to identify how Becky responded. Feeling out of control, she continued her inappropriate behavior, and the dance continued. Becky was struggling to gain trust, and the manager continued to focus her interventions on Step Two. She was no closer to her goals after 3 months. Where could this have ended? Like so many other cases, with Becky leaving the organization by choice or by being fired and definitely disgruntled.

Reviewing this with the manager, she understood how ineffective her actions had been. More importantly, she understood that she had never stopped to identify what she was trying to achieve. She was caught up in reacting. When she took the time to identify her goals, she realized that she wanted Becky to stop these behaviors and become a productive part of the team as she had been before.

When Becky did not respond positively, the manager should not have moved on to making requests. Instead, she should have recognized that Becky was not feeling in control. The manager needed to identify what interventions would help Becky regain control.

Remember, one of the most important functions when making requests is to provide feedback. People need this to ensure they are on the right track.

Step Three: Provide Transformational Coaching

They trust you, and your requests were clear and measurable. What next?

Step Three (Coach) is a time that you are able to connect with the individual with whom you are interacting. It is the best time to provide feedback. This is the exciting time for everyone, and this connection can be very productive. This is where individuals can grow and develop. Some would say this is when they change.

> **Coaching is the step where you connect with individuals. It is a step when defenses are reduced.**

Consider this: receiving criticism from anyone that you do not have a relationship with does not work. You will dismiss or avoid them. Once trust has been developed and a reasonable request has been made, individuals are more apt to listen to any suggestions you may have to improve what they are doing. Not everyone can handle constructive suggestions. This is why spending the majority of your energy on Steps One and Two will assist you in being successful at Step Three. By understanding others' personality styles and other aspects of their Circles of Control, you can identify the most effective manner in which to express this feedback. If you fail to present this criticism in a way they can hear it, you could erode their trust and find yourself back on step one attempting to build trust.

Providing constructive criticism is only half the work with this step. As individuals accept your suggestions, it is imperative that you support their efforts and successes. You must celebrate their achievements. This intervention is definitely the most missed step in health care today. We do not celebrate our own or others' achievements. Without doing this you cannot truly transform others' behaviors. They have to know you truly care for them. This encourages them to keep trying and believe in your support. These efforts will carry you to step four.

As I met with Becky, I was not sure if I would ever reach a point at which she would allow me to provide feedback, but I was able to encourage her to express herself and tell me what had occurred at work. She received my suggestions of how she could interpret others' statements and comments in a different manner. I made sure I provided feedback to her on her progress.

During the last 5 years, there has been a great deal written on coaching, mentoring, and transformation coaching. According to Kathy Malloch and Tim Porter-O'Grady, authors of *Quantum Leadership: A Textbook Of New Leadership*, transformational coaching involves developing a staff culture that focuses on outcomes and achievement, supporting autonomous and accountable staff behavior. Quite simply, with transformational coaching, staff are empowered and given the tools to manage their workplace and have a major role in the outcomes of their program. Transformational coaching requires that trust be built with staff for these principles to succeed. It also supports an atmosphere that encourages autonomy, control, and respect. Malloch and Porter-O'Grady state that "building trust is the key element into moving forward with transformational coaching." We will address the principles of transformational coaching in more detail in the fifth truth. What I want you to take from this is the connection between establishing trust and the ability to coach and change workplace cultures.

In the health care arena, this is called mentoring. Mentoring programs can be valuable for retention and recruitment. However, if this is done without taking steps one and two into consideration, the success of a mentoring program will be limited, especially when recruiting new graduates. Their sense of trust is minimal. They are fragile and do not have the experience to understand our world. Every coach and mentor needs to understand the Success Steps model in order for new hires to succeed. This applies to all staff: everyone needs coaching and at the right time.

Let us look at one more author who evaluates the connection between trust, being in control, and coaching.

Bob Adams, author of *Managing People*, states "Coaching is critical to managing the new work force. Coaching requires managers to direct employees by influencing not by controlling them. Effective coaching can boost morale and productivity tremendously by making employees feel empowered and by creating a feeling of ownership of their work." Much of what has been stated in the Success Steps model is supported by Bob Adams in his book. He understands not only the need to coach but the need for individuals to feel in control of their work environment. He goes on to say that "Coaching is based on influence and leadership and represents a management communication style that accepts employees as valuable and contributing individuals."

Managers struggle with coaching. It requires communication and active listening skills. Bob Adams further identifies the specific tips for managers in preparation for coaching.

1. Put in mind everything that is going on and focus on the session with the employee.
2. Define specifically what the coaching session will cover and the time it involves.

3. Inform the employee of the time and the place and the goals of the coaching session.
4. Be relaxed, cordial, and try to alleviate any perceived anxiety of the employee.

When you look back on these tips, you will see similarities to the guidelines of the Control Reaction Map. All of them are an attempt to help keep individuals in control.

Step Four: Achieve Goals

The last step is by far the most satisfying: Achieve Goals.

For today's health care professionals, this last step is often missing in their work. As a result of not experiencing this step, many decide to leave health care. In the first truth, you heard about a nurse who no longer hears the words "thank you" as frequently as she used to in her career. Unfortunately, this is all too common.

In addition to achieving your goal, you also get to experience a wonderful interaction with your patients. Patients at this fourth stage are able to step back and look at their behavior and apologize to you or, at best, identify how they treated you. This is a great experience that happens too infrequently. When it does occur with your patients, it motivates and reaffirms why you chose this profession. When it occurs with your peers and supervisors, it can be the reason you remain in your current position.

Becky said to me, "I am so sorry for the way I treated you. I am so glad you stuck with me and didn't turn away even when I was being rude." That's the reward of using the Success Steps principles. This story has a happy ending. Becky is still employed at the same hospital and working for the same manager. She reports that she has a whole new outlook on life and that her relationships at work (and at home) are much different.

The Success Steps, coupled with what you now know about personality styles, will enable you to influence the experiences and responses of others. All of this is essential not only when dealing with coworkers but also when managing difficult patients and their families, as we will discuss in the fourth truth. You have the foundation to be successful in managing difficult patients and families, as well as your peers.

Here is another example of using the Success Steps model to manage conflict in relationships.

Consider this: in your personal relationships, everyone has a specific personality style. The difference in styles can lead to disagreements. In some relationships, it becomes the issue that can lead to divorce. However, it does not have to be that way. This book is not dedicated to developing relationships at home, but the principles are centrally applicable to all relationships.

Identify your personality style and your partner's. Understand how each of you thinks and processes differently. I use this in my life every day. In particular, take note of concerns and pitfalls and what you can do about them.

My wife and I quickly realized we have vastly different styles. She is a processor, and I am a politician. I noticed the difference on our first date. I wanted our first date to be spontaneous, and she wanted it planned out. As you can imagine, it became a challenge each day until we began to understand these principles together. We learned to gain each other's trust by letting each other be in control. This has resulted in each of us feeling better about ourselves and our relationship.

A great example of the differences in our personality styles is found in the simple task of cleaning our house. As a true politician, I decide at the last moment it is time to clean the house thoroughly. I move like wildfire through the house in record time. This, of course, frustrates and confounds her. My wife wants the cleaning day to be planned and has an ordered, step-by-step way of accomplishing a thoroughly clean house.

My first reaction (feeling out of control) when this came up was to tell her she should be grateful that I was cleaning. (Obviously, this was not a good idea, and I don't recommend it.) You can probably guess what happened. My actions caused her reaction (feeling out of control)—to act out. She verbalized her displeasure with my statement.

As we both began to understand this dynamic, we began to understand that we were creating our own experiences and decided to make changes. We started learning about each other's styles and accepting each other for the way we were. We began laughing at each other's personality traits, which relieved a great deal of tension and stress. More importantly, we began to allow times in our lives to be unstructured and spontaneous, and I began allowing for structure in certain aspects of our lives. We both understood this was the first step to feeling safe in our relationship, to giving each other control. It paved the way for us to "make requests" (Step Two) of each other and honor those requests without being defensive.

Our communication channels expanded, and our relationship grew deeper. We began to offer suggestions to each other on how to handle different aspects of our lives (Step Three, Coach). This is when things really began to get good. Some would describe our relationship as a give-and-take relationship. We prefer to think of it as a "give-and-receive" relationship.

TRUTH #4:

SUCCESSFULLY CARING FOR DIFFICULT PEOPLE

Managing all Types of Patients and Families and Achieving Your Goals

The art of progress is to preserve order amid change.

—Alfred North Whitehead

You are the front line in this era of dramatic changes in health care. The responses from these changes can affect you in a variety of ways and from a variety of sources. These responses, in many instances, are unpleasant ones. They can include general rudeness, verbal and sexual abuse, and explosive or violent behavior. They can be caused by patients, families, peers, and supervisors. The complaints I hear from staff most often focus on patients and their families.

Without a doubt, this issue is the most frequently requested topic for discussion from nurses and health care personnel at my seminars throughout the country. Staff want to know how to deal with the patient and/or family that is difficult or uncooperative. For some, it has become the central reason for leaving the profession. For others, it is one of the primary sources of ongoing frustration. One nurse I spoke with described each day of work as a battle. She found herself under constant scrutiny by her patients and families. She told me, "Every day we move so fast that patients and their families feel this pace and react to it because it scares them. I guess they feel they have to protect themselves and their loved ones to assure they are getting the best care. The entire situation is just so frustrating for all of us."

Other nurses have told me they believe patients and families act out because they feel out of control. It stems from fear: fear of how sick they are, fear of the pace at which we move, and fear of the unknown. Quite simply, they are scared.

Recall the dynamics we discussed in the first truth. All these external dynamics (shorter length of stay, shortages of staff, technology, etc.) contribute to the defensive nature of everyone. According to Doris Heldge, PhD, in her article "Turning Workplace Anger into Peak Performance," we have programmed customers and patients into a consumer-focused group. This has created more vocal and difficult individuals. They can be harder to satisfy. At some level we can understand their responses, but what is the impact on you?

It can be devastating. Not hearing the words "thank you," as well as hearing increasing complaints and criticisms, is taking its toll on all of you. This environment directly affects your level of satisfaction. After all, who wants to come to work each day to be yelled at or demeaned?

The complaints about this issue seem to continue to grow. Jeanette Erickson, one of the authors of the article "The Nursing Shortage: Solutions for the Short and Long Term," stated, "The retention of nurses begins with how the organization does or does not value the staff." Staff look to see how management supports them with difficult patients and families. Erickson goes on to say that professional respect is central in nurses' decisions to remain in their profession. This includes respect from patients and their families as well.

These trends provide a potentially dangerous experience for health care workers. Both of these examples identify difficult environments in which to work. Let's explore what happens to you as you are affected by this world and begin to "protect" yourself.

Frequent experience dealing with difficult and explosive patients and families can lead you to feel out of control. This is your way of coping, not who you are. You deal with the difficult patients by avoiding them. Some of you react (act out), yelling at families that you perceive to be taking away your control or attacking your identity.

If you do not think this happens, observe your peers next time you are at work. They are not immune to responding positively or negatively to patients. In many cases, they act out and socialize negatively, keeping themselves from moving beyond step one. They continue to create this experience and then complain that they are unhappy. What is wrong with this picture?

They have a choice. They do not have to experience growing frustration and anger. This is what I want you to learn about yourself and your world. *You* choose your experience. Yes, events outside your control do happen, people do act in less than ideal ways, and yet you still get to choose your own response. You are not helpless, nor are you a victim. Before we can move forward with this chapter, you have to agree with this.

Please stop and think about how you respond to these situations at work. Notice how you choose to respond. What would happen if you reacted in a different way?

Using the Success Steps model you can empower yourself to manage these types of patients and families (and for that matter, anyone in your life). All you have to do is say, "I am in control of my own experience, and these tools will assist me in realizing this." Without living life consciously, you can find yourself in a vicious cycle. You become angrier, and your behaviors become magnified, spiraling you more and more out of control. For many, they leave their jobs only to repeat this experience at another job or in a different career.

So where do you fit in this description? Are you aware of your ability to choose your experience, or are you merely letting your environment control your actions by living life unconsciously? Chances are you already know. You picked up this book for a reason. You may even find yourself nodding in agreement as you read these chapters or even highlighting or making notes on sections that seem particularly relevant to you. You can study the concepts presented so far in light of stress factors.

Let's get down to business. How does the Circle of Control relate to your experiences at work? Look back at the personal Circle of Control you created in Truth #2. Are you aware of your specific self-worth list? Does anything on your list interfere with your interactions with patients and families? Have they said anything that hits too close to home?

For example, if your number one priority is to be a parent but your reality is that work takes priority over everything else, you will become frustrated, possibly projecting this frustration to your patients and families. Or, you may overreact if a patient says something like, "You can't even take care of me; I'll bet you're a terrible parent." Believe it or not, this is an actual statement a nurse from Denver shared with me at a conference. This nurse made a decision to leave nursing after this experience but came to the conference because she had already registered. After we spoke for over an hour, she had a different outlook on her experience. She understood why she reacted in the manner she did and understood how to create a new experience. This holds true for patients and families as well.

What about your personality style? How does this play into your ability to manage difficult and explosive personalities? Not being aware of your style or the style of your patients and/or their families and how that relates to the Control Reaction Map can be detrimental. Pointers and processors want to direct and take control. Patients and families who already feel out of control may feel more so. Taking control is okay, but not to the point of preventing your patient from having some sense of control. Politicians and peacemakers do not have a need to be in control, but some patients and families react to their lack of direction. Without clear expectations and structure, they can begin to feel out of control as well.

Do you find it interesting that I have begun this truth of managing difficult patients and families by looking at you? You shouldn't. What you bring to work (Circle of Control) will set the tone with your patients and families. You have to be conscious of your own Circle of Control before you can successfully care for difficult patients and their families.

As we discussed in truth two, we know that under stress the dominant personality style will surface and present itself to you. In the second aspect of the Control Reaction Map (page 44), patients and families will bring their perceived experiences as well as their past experiences to your interaction. Now, I don't know about you, but somewhere along the line, most family members and patients have not had a positive experience in a hospital setting. It is very likely that they will project these past experiences. It is very important for you to be aware of this and to be ready for their reaction.

The third aspect is the communication patterns. Individuals who are stressed and overwhelmed will express their stress through their verbal and nonverbal interactions. If they are feeling out of control, they will avoid you, ignore you, and be very short in their responses to your questions. Please refer to the third truth to review verbal and nonverbal responses.

Helping Patients and Families to Regain Control

Now that we have an understanding of why a patient or family may feel out of control, how do we use the Success Steps model to assist them in regaining their control?

Let's refer to the establishment of structure and boundaries in Step One of the Success Steps model. Remember, in the third truth, we discussed how important structure and boundaries can be in developing a sense of self for individuals. We have also have learned from the Control Reaction Map that a consistent feeling of being out of control can lead to decreased sense of self. Clear structure and boundaries for patients places them in a better position to be in control. They need to understand what you expect of them. This may need to be presented to them in a different manner based on their personality style.

When I had asked families and patients who have been out of control and subsequently have regained control what it is they were experiencing, they will tell me a lack of understanding of what was happening to them and what they could do to manage their lives (be in control). At that moment, they could not say it, but this is what they were experiencing. I am sure this is consistent among patients and families.

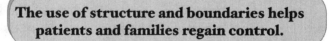

The use of structure and boundaries helps patients and families regain control.

Let's look at an example of using structure to help a patient and family regain control. First, you have to determine if they are demonstrating out-of-control behavior. By asking open-ended questions such as "What do you need?" or "How can I help you?" the difficult patient will either respond by avoiding you or making a negative comment such as "If you don't know, who does?" or "Am I supposed to do everything?" Once you have determined this, providing structure can allow them an understanding of what to do to succeed.

What you are doing is simply putting more structure around an individual who continues to act out. This is not in the form of controlling any individual; it's in the form of placing patients and their families in a place to succeed. If your open-ended question (just described) is met with more anger and frustration, redirect your question to what you need from them at that moment. For example, "Mr. Smith, for the next 20 minutes this is the procedure that I will be doing, and during that time, I need you to follow my directions." If you get a positive response, meaning that they agree with what you are doing, then you can move forward. You have placed them in a position of control. If, indeed, they continue to act out, you need to provide additional structure and boundaries for them, again, to put them in place to succeed, not to be controlling. This may be as specific to that moment as how you need them positioned, what the family can do, or what is going to occur in the next 5 minutes.

I hope that you are starting to get a sense that as I am dealing with a more difficult patient, I provide more structure to help them achieve. Many of you are saying, "You want me to continue to press an angry individual who does not want my care?" That is not what I am saying. If someone requests to be left alone and not be managed, then I am going to honor that request. However, if the interactions (verbal and nonverbal) continue to go on and the patient or family wants me to be a part of that interaction, I am going to place them in a position to succeed. There is a very clear difference.

We understand how patients and their families react when they are stressed and feel angry, but how does this affect you and how do you respond? During my interviews with nurses, most stated their most common coping strategy is avoidance. They hope by ignoring these types of patients that the problem will go away and there will be no conflict. You now know this is not correct, and it does not work. You understand that everyone wants to feel in control, including you. If you are unaware of the Control Reaction Map, you could find yourself feeling out of control and acting out yourself. What does this look like? It can range from avoidance to rude remarks to patients and families.

Consider some of your most difficult patients. You were rarely able to avoid them. They still found ways to interact with you in order to take control; it just happened to be an unpleasant experience. Maybe the call light went on more than those of other patients. Maybe their needs remained unmet or their pain was never in control. Whatever the reason, their out-of-control behavior can prompt your out-of-control behavior-producing outcomes, poor patient and family satisfaction, poor care outcomes, and poor staff satisfaction. And, of course, your professional relationship remains on step one, waiting for trust to be initiated.

Let's look at a story to better illustrate this dynamic. This is a story about Mary, a nurse on an adult general med/surge unit from Indianapolis, who was experienced and confident in her ability to manage even the most difficult patients, or so she thought...

It didn't take long for Mary to know that this wasn't going to be like her other 12-hour shifts. From the look on her coworkers' faces and the volume on the board, she knew this was going to be one of those nights. She wasn't worried, though. She had faced this for the last 3 years and felt confident she could manage whatever was sent her way.

As she sat down to report, she quickly learned they were once again short staffed, a common experience to which she had become accustomed. She was assigned three patients, one intubated on the ventilator and sedated on an ativan drip. Her second patient had just been downgraded; however, she was told it would be difficult finding her a medical bed. Her third patient, 55-year-old John, had been admitted with DKA (diabetic ketoacidosis), was insulin dependent, and had been noncompliant with his treatment regimen. As a result, he was on his fourth admission in the last year. The day shift nurse reported that he had a history of hypertension and alcohol abuse, drinking a six-pack daily. She also described John as belligerent, refusing routine meds and threatening to go to the AMA. He was verbally abusive, yelling obscenities at the staff, and had twice pulled out his IV. His call light went off regularly, and many of the times that she entered the room there was no specific reason for the call.

Mary took the information and didn't think too much of it. She prided herself on the ability to handle all kinds of patients, and she thought that this would not be any different for her. On entering John's room, Mary was greeted with a cold stare and a nonverbal patient. She began to introduce herself and received no response. She explained to him what she would be doing during that shift and began with her assessment. During her instructions, he did not answer her. However, as she began to take vital signs, he screamed and yelled at her, "What the hell are you doing?" She looked at him and stated, "I was just taking your vitals." He stated, "Who are you? You come into the room; you talk nonstop, and then just begin to work on me. There are so many people in and out of this room, how do you expect me to get better?" Mary began to apologize and tried to explain again what she was doing. He became more agitated and asked her to leave. "Get the hell out! I don't need this; I don't need you in here doing whatever you're doing. I just want to go to sleep." Mary froze. No patient had ever talked to her in this manner. She did not know what to do. He yelled again. "Didn't you hear me?" Without much thought, she turned around and left the room. She went behind the nurse's station and just stared at the wall. She wasn't sure what she should do next.

Shortly after this she found herself getting angry and frustrated that somebody would treat her in that manner. She had dealt with difficult families before, but there always seemed to be a good reason for their anger, and she usually was able to find a way to put them in a better mood. She had never been kicked out of a room and told not to come back and wondered what to do. Should she tell anyone? She hesitated to do this because she has always had a reputation for managing all kinds of patients. Should she try to avoid him? Should she just ignore it and go on? She felt embarrassed.

Thirty-five minutes later, Mary knocked on the door again and found John awake and asked if she could come in to set up his medications. He mumbled, "OK, but no talking. Just do what you have to do and get out!" So she began to set the medications. She found she could not help herself and had to ask him why he was so angry with her. As soon as she began to question this, John became more and more frustrated and stated, "All I asked you to do was to give me my meds and not talk about anything else. What are you, stupid?" At that point, Mary shut down, gathered her supplies, and left the room.

Can you relate to this kind of patient?

In my interviews, I was told many stories like this one. In nearly all these cases, the primary strategy used was avoidance: avoidance of uncomfortable situations and potential explosions. The problem, of course, is that it never works. Nurses who left their profession spoke openly to me about not feeling appreciated and having too many of these kinds of patients. Mary was always the kind of nurse that her peers would turn to when there was someone difficult to handle because she had a certain approach about her that decreased people's defenses, but in this case, she couldn't understand why she wasn't received well and why the patient was so angry. The more that she pressed, the more frustrated he became. She told me that she found herself not knowing what to do, what to say, or how to involve the patient in the treatment again.

Later, she told me this is who she is: "I am an outgoing individual who is usually able to win people over just by speaking with them." When I asked her about personality styles and different approaches to winning people over, she told me that she had never heard how this could help her. As I began to explain the 4-P Personality Styles and the Success Steps model, her eyes grew wide and she began nodding with each explanation.

To be successful caring for John, Mary realized she needed to understand her Circle of Control and began implementing the Success Steps model. Her understanding of her Circle of Control would have helped her avoid reacting negatively to John's behavior. In fact, these principles work in reverse as well. Suddenly Mary begins to feel out of control. She begins to withdraw from the client, becomes angry and possibly rude to him. The results are the same. She never gets beyond step one, and her experience is not a positive one.

Initially, Mary should have realized that she was dealing with an angry individual. As we know from the Success Steps model, she had not initially developed a sense of trust with John, and he was feeling out of control. He was expressing this lack of control by being belligerent and refusing direction. He was also determined to structure his social interaction with Mary in a negative manner as evident by his repeated call lights.

So what should Mary have done to achieve the outcome she wanted? First, she needed to understand her own Circle of Control and her personality style, along with John's. Doing this she would have realized that she is a peacemaker and has adopted a style of using her sense of humor and kindness to avoid conflict. This has usually worked for her, but because she was interacting with a pointer, her techniques were not successful. It has been my experience that angry pointers appear to feel more out of control when they are interacting with others who do not provide clear direction.

Second, she needed to depersonalize his behavior, not take it personally. By understanding the first step in the Success Steps and why he was expressing himself in this manner, Mary could recognize John's out-of-control behavior and respond more effectively to obtain trust.

Third, she needed to give some time for him to feel that he was in control of his world. When John finally let her in to set up the medications, he specifically stated exactly what he wanted done, and Mary should have followed that explicitly. By trying to receive additional information against his requests, Mary again lost John's trust.

Phrases that Mary should have used when speaking with John, and which would be more to the liking of somebody who feels out of control, are "What do you need?" and "What can I do for you?" Based on the response of the client, it is imperative to repeat back exactly what they said to make sure both of you are clear on the direction. This sense of structure and established boundaries can place John in a position to be in control. Remember our discussion of setting boundaries and providing clearer direction to provide the patient with a better sense of control. This can initiate the process of trust. In fact, patients like John have such a difficult time interacting with others that they may request to work with only you in the future.

After meeting with Mary and reviewing these techniques, she agreed and understood that once the client started to express himself in an angry manner, she lost all sight of her goals and immediately began to react, feeling out of control and angry herself.

As you can tell by the story with Mary, dealing with difficult and explosive personalities is by far one of the greatest challenges that nurses and other health care personnel face today. When you speak with people, they describe it as "uncomfortable." They would rather not deal with conflict or avoid a situation that might create conflict. If you have learned anything, it is that you cannot avoid conflict. All you can do is help people feel in control, reducing the conflictual situation and emotions. Through avoidance, which is the most common strategy health care professionals use, you begin to promote out-of-control behavior, and it is the catalyst that directs people to respond to you in an adversarial way. Once somebody begins to be angry or out of control, there are specific steps that you can take to de-escalate the situation and refocus him or her to the issue at hand. These techniques empower people to take control of their behavior.

Following are the top 10 techniques for managing difficult patients and their families. Each of these steps is sequential in nature and supports the Success Steps model.

1. Before entering into an interaction, review all aspects of the situation.
2. Clearly introduce yourself and the purpose for meeting. This sets clear boundaries and expectations.
3. Identify a quiet area conducive to discussing the situation without being interrupted.

4. Encourage and allow individuals to fully explain their interpretation of the issue at hand.
5. While this is occurring, determine personality style. You will get clues from the words people use as well as their interpretation of events.
6. Give them control. Do not get defensive.
7. Once they have explained the situation attempt to identify a mutual goal. Remember, speak to them in a way their personality style can hear you.
8. Identify all agreed-on actions and make sure they are measurable.
9. Identify how feedback should be provided.
10. Celebrate the achievement of the goal.

Carefully evaluate these 10 techniques. Let's take some time to review them. Before you enter into any situation, really take the time to understand all the issues. This means, not only your perception of the situation, but others' as well. Attempt to get a complete and accurate synopsis of the situation. Once you have completed this and you have approached the patient or families that you need to meet with, introduce yourself, your position, and what your role is in their care. This intervention begins the process of setting boundaries and structure in your professional relationship with your patient and your family.

Find a quiet area that reduces the amount of noise and distraction for your conversation. You also want to avoid having this discussion in front of other people. This will only cause people to be more defensive. Clearly articulate what your concern is and then allow the patient and/or family to explain their interpretation of the issue. Don't interrupt them, don't react to them, just listen. It can also be very helpful to write down the specific issues as they speak. This demonstrates to them your willingness to understand their specific issues and provides a sense of confidence and control.

As they begin to explain their version of the situation, determine their personality style. Refer back to the third truth, which will assist you.

Throughout this process, continue to let them maintain control, and do not get defensive. Once the situation has been reviewed by both of you, begin to identify common goals that you want to achieve. Remember, speak to individuals in a way their personality style will hear you best.

After both of you have determined agreed-on goals, begin to identify the steps that will occur to reach this goal. You are doing this to create a mechanism to keep both of you on track to reaching the goal. Make these steps measurable. If anything is subjective, conflict can continue to arise because it's one person's word against another whether you actually achieved this step. You are going to have to determine how often you're going to meet or review these action steps. Make sure that you set times to review the progress toward these goals. When both parties have achieved the desired goal, celebrate this. I am not talking about having a party, but I am speaking about acknowledging the accomplishment and the effort that the patient or the family has made. This is something that I will review further in the upcoming truths regarding how we as a profession do not celebrate our own achievements.

Here is another case study using these 10 techniques. Joe was going to be a first-time father. He wasn't sure what to expect. His full concern was on his wife and her comfort. When he entered the room, he was greeted with a loud moan from his wife, Sarah. She told him that the pain was really becoming unbearable and asked Joe to find a doctor to give her a shot. Joe left the room and went to the nurse's station where he saw a woman leaning over the desk writing feverishly. He remembered this vividly because he couldn't get out of his mind the vision of her rapidly chewing gum as he walked towards her. Joe waited momentarily as he stood at the desk, but the nurse gave no indication that she knew he was there. Joe said, "Excuse me." The nurse, without looking up, put her finger in the air and said, "Wait a minute, sir." She continued to write and, as Joe noticed, chew her gum.

Joe could hear his wife still moaning in pain because the room was adjacent to the nurse's station. Despite this, he patiently waited and once again asked the nurse to speak with him. Because he got no response, Joe became more and more agitated. He placed his open hand on the desk and, apparently without realizing it, made a thudding sound. The nurse was so startled that she jumped back and looked at Joe and said, "Now sir, just relax. I don't know why you are so angry." On hearing this, Joe became even more frustrated and said, "Angry? I am not angry; I am just trying to get your attention." Again the nurse replied, "Just relax sir; you're getting upset." At this, Joe said, "All I want to do is speak to you, and you keep ignoring me. My wife is in pain, and I need some assistance. Then the nurse said, "Relax," backed up further, and went into the conference room. Very frustrated, Joe waited patiently for her to return. About 2 minutes later, the nurse came out with the supervisor, who approached Joe with her arms folded and said, "What seems to be the problem, sir?" Joe attempted to explain the situation to the supervisor, who continued to address him from behind the desk with her arms folded. As Joe began describing what had occurred, he continued to hear his wife in the adjacent room, moaning louder. He said, "I don't have time to sit here and explain this to you. Can you just please have the physician..." and before he could finish his sentence, the supervisor stated, "Sir, you need to calm down. We know what we are doing. We will get the proper care for you and your wife." Frustrated, Joe quickly turned around and said, "I can't believe you people" and went back into his wife's room.

Joe told me he remembers this next part of the story very clearly because it was roughly 3:30 pm, and he wasn't expecting the response from the staff he was about to receive. Joe, at this point, was extremely angry and was ready to get anyone he needed to get some treatment for his wife. As he approached the desk, his arms were now folded. He was determined not to take "no" for an answer and to become louder if necessary. The first thing he noticed was that it wasn't the same nurse that he was speaking to earlier. He very clearly and abruptly stated, "I would like to speak with the nurse who is taking care of my wife in room 238." Very calmly and very slowly, the nurse behind the desk put her pen down, looked up and stood up, and stated, "You must be Mr. Teller." She immediately reached out her hand to shake his and said, "Very nice to meet you. I am the nurse in charge of your wife this evening." Joe, stunned by the pleasant tone, smile, and friendliness, hesitated but eventually shook her hand. Before anything else was said, the nurse, Joan, asked Joe if she could speak with him. Not sure what she wanted to speak about he said, "Yes." She came out from behind the desk and asked Joe if they could meet in a quieter area, walked with him to a vacant seating area, sat down, leaned in towards Joe, and said, "I know there have been some problems with the first shift, and I am not sure of everything that occurred. I am, however, concerned with how I can help you at this time. Would you please tell me what the issues are and how I can assist you and your wife?"

Joe, still not sure of Joan's motives, quickly continued in his defensive mode (his arms folded and leaning away from the nurse) and began talking about his experience with the first-shift nurse and how his wife was still in pain. Joan listened and did not interrupt.

When Joe was finished she said, "Thank you for explaining to me what had happened. I am sorry you had a bad experience." Joe became very much at ease after his initial conversation with Joan. He unfolded his arms, leaned back, and was very pleased.

Joan then looked at Joe and said, "I need your assistance. I am not sure how much you know and don't know, and I don't want to presume what level of knowledge you have." Joe nodded and laughed and said, "Well, I know there is a baby, I know it is coming out, everything else in-between is kind of foggy." Both began to laugh, and Joan thanked Joe again for his candor and honesty. She explained exactly what the next 4 to 5 hours would entail. She then gave him very specific directions, instruction about what she was going to do and what she needed him to do. "As soon as we are done, I will walk over and page the physician to make sure that your wife's pain will be taken care of. Once I have completed that, there are a couple of things you can do to help your wife relax." Joan began to explain to Joe some massage techniques and how to use ice chips and cool washcloths. When they finished the conversation (which took only 6 minutes), Joan reviewed the goals again with Joe. Both agreed, and Joan told him once the physician had been in the room and completed his work, she would follow up with Joe to see how he was doing on the assignments she had given him.

True to form, within 20 minutes, the physician came, Joe's wife's pain had ceased, and Joe began implementing the procedures given to him by Joan. Twenty minutes after that, like clockwork, Joan came in and began to view Joe's interventions with his wife. She immediately gave him some positive feedback about how well he was doing and continued to laugh and joke with both of them. Joan looked at Joe's wife and said, "I am glad your pain is better, and I am glad your husband was so helpful in making you feel more comfortable." Both Joe and his wife thanked Joan for her care.

Joan did a wonderful job, not only meeting the needs of a patient but also de-escalating an angry and frustrated family member and achieved her identified goals (as well as Joe's). Joan clearly walked through all 10 steps of the techniques for returning control, creating an atmosphere in which the patient's family was in control, patient care outcomes were reached, and conflict was minimized.

When the next shift began, the charge nurse and the day-shift nurse began to complain about Joe and how difficult he was to work with. It even went so far that they all were trying to avoid taking him as a patient during the assignment. Joan spoke up immediately and

said that she would be glad to work with him and asked her colleagues to explain everything that had occurred. As the charge
nurse and day nurse began to explain the situation, they focused
only on Joe's behavior, not their own role in the escalation. Joan
asked for clarification of the facts. She also asked them what they
did in response to his behavior. They couldn't answer. They could
not explain why they reacted the way they did.

What about Joan? What worked for her? Why was she successful
where her colleagues were not?

Let's look at each of her steps. Once she had all the facts from her
colleagues, she approached Joe, introduced herself, and asked to
talk in a quieter area. Joan carefully listened to Joe's explanation of
the situation, not becoming defensive, not disagreeing, and not
cutting him off. Joan wasn't sure exactly what personality style she
was dealing with but continued providing him the ability to feel in
control and, by listening to him, to feel better about himself. As Joe
finished his explanations, Joan was able to identify a common goal
that was measurable and time limited. The follow through on all her
promises and requests to Joe was wonderful. I cannot emphasize
this enough: if you do not follow through on your promises, you will
erode any trust that has been developed, and you will remain on
step one.

Do you see how this works? Joan's behavior was exemplary. In
fact, by using these techniques for returning control, Joan was able
to achieve her clinical goals, help the patient and family be in
control, and do it in less time than she would have by using avoidance and conflict interaction. These techniques work and, as you
use them, you will find that you become more efficient and effective, taking less time overall. Some nurses have said to me, "I don't
have time for all these steps." If managing difficult patients and
their families is one of the biggest causes of nurse burnout and at-
trition, as the research indicates, do you really have time *not* to use
these techniques? By following the de-escalation steps, the principles of the Control Reaction Map, and Success Steps, you will save
yourself time and aggravation. You will also create a rewarding experience for you, your patients, and their families.

TRUTH #5:

MANAGING DIFFICULT COWORKERS AND SUPERVISORS

Believe It or Not, Not Everyone Gets Along.

The reason most major goals are not achieved is that we spend our time doing second things first.

—*Robert J. McKain*

As much as I have talked to you about how popular discussing difficult patients and families in my seminars has been, the opposite is true for this next truth. Rarely do I get questions regarding the relationships among coworkers, especially when it comes to conflict and getting along. However, it is after my seminars that I receive a lot of questions in this area. It is a very emotional topic for many health care professionals. They do not feel comfortable sharing these issues, but they need to discuss them with someone.

This makes sense, doesn't it? There can be some level of rationalization when a patient or family is difficult to work with because there is something in the back of your head that supplies the reason for the behavior, and you are able to understand on some level. When it comes to your peers, people that you work with every day, it is not the same issue. There is an emotional connection, and their comments feel more personal to us.

I have to tell you that in my interviews with nurses, the first topic that is raised is the issue of people with whom they work. Ask people to stay and work overtime, and tell me what their first response is. You've got it; they want to know who their coworkers will be. In fact, I have talked with nurses who have told me that they would choose to work short-handed with the peers of their choice than be overstaffed with individuals with whom they have conflicts.

This is a powerful statement and expression from nurses who hold patient safety in such high regard. Nurses see a clear connection between team cohesiveness and patient care. According to Sandra Thomas and Patricia Droppleman, authors of an article, "Channeling Nurses' Anger into Positive Interventions," nurses who have minimal conflict or have an active process for dealing with conflict have higher patient service outcomes. She also goes on to state that organizations with a culture that is supportive of addressing staff conflicts or issues on a shift-by-shift basis are much healthier groups.

In fact, without even reviewing the most up-to-date research in the area of staff conflict and concerns, it is common sense that the atmosphere for delivering great patient care is enhanced if the team is cohesive and has active conflict management skills.

> **Patient care is enhanced when team cohesiveness and active conflict management skills exist.**

Let's review studies identifying causes of workplace conflict.

In 1995, Cullen, author of "Burnout: Why Do We Blame the Nurse?" identified several factors that can create a toxic environment and fuel nurses' anger.

1. Multiple regulations of mandates and reimbursement issues in the health care system
2. Structural and environmental factors in the institutional system (short staffing, insufficient supplies and equipment, demands for nurses to lower patient care standards to cut costs)
3. Devaluation of nursing work by the societal system
4. Poor preparation of nurses with regard to being proactive in the extraordinary situations they face

Carlson-Catalono, in a large national study in a 1990 report, learned that nurses perceive their work environment as constraining. They report that these constraints impede physical needs, personal needs, and professional needs, making them feel powerless.

Further research by Stokols in 1992 described "conflict-prone organizations that are characterized by the presence of rigid ideologies, non-participatory organizational processes, absence of shared goals, and existence of competitive coalitions and prospects of unemployment stemming from economic changes." He further stated that nurses can recognize these qualities in their organization and have a very good understanding of why conflict is occurring. His research identified that "conflict can erupt at any time but is most prevalent during periods of rapid environmental and social change."

Lastly, in 1995 Davies contended that without a system that includes nurses and policy development, program review, and partnerships with other clinical personnel, conflict can continue to rise as a result of feeling out of control.

Now this sounds familiar. As we embark on the Control Reaction Map and the Success Steps, the research clearly focuses on the lack of control, which can contribute to conflictual situations in the workplace. Doesn't it seem as if we have heard these issues before? These are further examples of external factors that affect all of you, causing a reaction. This is usually a feeling of being out of control, but remember, it doesn't have to be this way.

Let's look at more studies. A study by Hillhouse and Addler (in press) found that nurses with the highest burnout scores and the highest levels of affective and physical symptoms were ones who had conflict with other nurses and supervisors.

J. A. Rodgers, in 1982, established a theory of why envy among nurses results in interpersonal clashes. The research dates the origin of human envy to the early exclusive relationship of the infant with the mother. It identifies the breast as the first object of envy and, by extension, the woman is therefore the first person envied. Rogers points out that "nursing, being a predominantly female occupation, conjures up the image of the nursing mother. Therefore, the profession is 'vulnerable' to angry, envious, destructive, though perhaps large in conscious, impulses of the many others with whom we deal—patients as well as physicians as well as other colleagues."

According to Thomas and Droppleman, several factors can contribute to interpersonal discord.

1. Unfair, uncivil treatment
2. Gender discrimination

3. Irresponsibility of ancillary personnel
4. Turf battles over what part of the patient is the doctor's and what is the nurse's
5. Physical conditions such as noise, congestion, and uncomfortable temperatures
6. Unavoidable physical proximity of conflicted individuals

In fact, subsequent studies identified a continual conflict regarding the hierarchal doctor–nurse relationship. In their research, nurses said doctors use them as "scapegoats" and "whipping posts," and they described tirades and being "lambasted, thrashed, picked on, belittled, and lectured." The authors went on to say that this research was duplicated in 1995 by Manderino and Berkey who validate their findings. In their sample, they reviewed 130 nurses, and 90% had experienced verbal abuse from physicians during the past year. They further evaluated the response of nurses to this abuse, and in their research, they found that of the 130 participants, 45%, as well as 45% of all health care personnel, were victims of abuse during childhood themselves thus being in an abusive situation again.

Thomas and Droppleman provided a poem in their research that they obtained from an article from Kalisch and Kalisch (1977).

Nurses moving quietly,

Voices hushed in awe,

All things silent waiting,

Obedient to the law.

That we have heard so often,

But I'll repeat once more:

All things must be in order

When doctors are on the floor.

Additional conflictual issues occur as a result of the anger nurses have towards supervisory personnel. They further found that what made the nurses angry was "authoritarian, fault-finding and uncaring behavior." We will further evaluate this area in the next truth.

The last findings in Thomas and Droppleman's research were in the area of "horizontal violence." Participants described hostile interactions among nurses in graphic terms, i.e., needling, cutting, blasting, and backbiting to name a few. The term "horizontal violence" was identified by Muff in 1982, along with its behavior, characteristic of oppressed groups, who, unable to effectively retaliate against members of the dominant group (physicians, administrators, and supervisors), fight among each other instead. Their research identifies that the horizontal violence is not always overt; it can be very subtle.

I have provided you with multiple research articles dealing with conflicts and potential violence among nursing staff, and I would like to summarize this to help you understand exactly what all of this means. What follows is a list of what research studies have identified as causing conflict in the workplace for nurses and other health care professionals.

- Multiple accreditation regulations
- Staffing issues, including the mix of care personnel
- Devaluation of the role of the nurse
- Lack of nursing leadership during these stressful times
- Decreased flexibility
- Rapid workplace change
- Lack of conflict management skills
- Human envy
- Unfair, uncivil treatment
- Gender discrimination
- Physical proximity of conflicted individuals
- Nurse–doctor hierarchal dynamic
- Horizontal violence philosophy

Take a good look at this list. Do you find yourself identifying with any of these dynamics? The list is quite extensive. These areas were identified by you, and they are real. It does feel overwhelming. My intention is not to bore you with a litany of research articles depicting what other nurses think, but I truly believe that, with this truth, it is important to understand your reality. Issues in the health care workplace are unique and different from those in any other workplace setting.

So how does all this fit into our previous truths? According to the Control Reaction Map, you can see that conflict in the workplace can cause individuals to feel out of control. We know that when people feel out of control, they act out. This behavior will continue if the conflictual issues are not addressed.

How does conflict affect the Success Steps model? In a constant state of conflict, you remain on step one, trying to establish trust. It seems complex to address all these issues in order to develop trust, but it can be done, and we will show you how.

We understand that there is a relationship between conflict and anger. It is not going to go away, and it has to be managed appropriately. This is important in understanding anger. It does not just go away. Anger must be expressed. If you ignore anger, it will be expressed unconsciously in the form of unexpected outbursts, physical aches and pains, and complaints, to name a few.

Let's look at some of the top guidelines for managing your anger and avoiding conflict.

1. Acknowledge the moment that you are feeling angry and understand there is a source of this anger.
2. Return to your Circle of Control and evaluate the connection between your personality style and your specific self-worth as they relate to the conflict and anger.
3. Talk to someone in your external support system about the anger you are feeling. Do not keep this information inside. Determine the cause of your conflict.
4. Determine if the expectations regarding your conflict are realistic or unrealistic.
5. Identify the triggers to your conflict.
6. If the cause of the conflict is an individual at work, meet with that person to express your concerns. (Follow the conflict meeting guidelines in Truth #4.)
7. Evaluate your diet. Don't use excess food or alcohol to cope with the conflict.
8. Exercise regularly: walk, stretch, run. Get your blood flowing.
9. Meditate: find 15–20 minutes of down time to stop thinking and just be.
10. Leave work at work. It is not your home life.

These guidelines are comprehensive and are meant to help you take care of yourself. It all begins when you acknowledge when anger is present within yourself. Surprising as that may be, some of you are not connected to yourselves enough to be able to identify your anger. Once you have done this, now return to your Circle of Control. Start with yourself first; understand your personality style and your specific self-worth. Is there conflict that you can identify in these areas? Is the source of the stress and conflict that you are having with certain individuals related to your Circle of Control? This is the soul searching that you need to complete in order to establish the connection between stress in your life and the conflict you are experiencing.

> **Understanding who you are is the first step to managing your anger and avoiding conflict.**

This is when you need to use your external support system. Pull them off to the side, talk with them about what you are experiencing and get their take on the situation. Remember, they know you best. They understand your personality style and your specific self-worth.

Sometimes our expectations with regard to people and situations are not realistic. For example, I spoke with a nurse who told me that she didn't understand the need for conflict management skills because she doesn't experience conflict in her life. I told her that her expectations were unrealistic and that, despite her best intentions, conflict will occur in the work setting.

In another situation, a nursing supervisor told me that she expects everyone to follow her direction without question. My response to her was that this was unrealistic, and, based on the complexity of work settings and individuals, conflict will continue to occur.

Know what triggers your conflict. Your specific self-worth is a good start to understanding what specific triggers cause you to feel uncomfortable and stressed, but there might be others as well. Review your personality style. Recognize that there are certain characteristics in other personality styles that might cause you frustration and anger.

The sixth step involves addressing conflict with the conflict meeting guidelines. The only point I want to make here is that addressing conflict with anyone can be an extremely emotional experience.

The next three guidelines focus on nutrition, exercise, and the use of meditation. Your body has to be taken care of for you to manage the stress and conflict that will occur in your life. There are many wonderful books that talk about diet and exercise. I encourage you to create your own individualized plan for reaching optimal health. Strategies such as meditation and yoga, among others, can be extremely helpful for learning to create a sense of peace and a new experience for yourself.

The last guideline is to separate your work world from your home world. Establishing these boundaries is extremely important in preventing your work world from affecting your home life.

The purpose of these guidelines is to help you recognize and understand the source of your conflict and provide you with steps to reduce your stress. Remember, when we talked about the number one coping strategy that nurses use to deal with difficult patients and families, it was avoidance. It is not different in this scenario, but as we know, avoidance will not alleviate the conflict or your stress.

Managing Conflict

How do we alleviate the conflict? We do this by identifying the source of the conflict. If it is an individual, you need to address the issue with that person directly. For most of you, this could be the scariest intervention you've ever done. Confronting people about a certain behavior is not a popular thing to do. With 60% of health care workers being peacemakers, managing conflict is very uncomfortable. However, without addressing the conflictual situation, it worsens and the anger intensifies, affecting your ability to function at work and, eventually, if not addressed, causing burnout.

Let's review how we successfully manage a conflictual situation with the techniques for returning control (see Truth #4, page 68).

Before entering into this conversation, take the time to understand the entire situation. You certainly don't want to have an accusatory approach. Having all the facts will provide you with a sense of confidence. This intervention in and of itself causes a great deal of stress for many. Practice with someone ahead of time to reduce your anxiety. Meet with the individual in an area that is conducive for a discussion and free of interruption. Clearly identify why you are meeting and articulate this using only the facts. Avoid using subjective information; use only what actually has occurred. Let me further clarify this. When you speak to an individual about a specific situation, speak only in "I" statements.

> I need to speak with you, Bob, to talk about what occurred yesterday outside Mr. Smith's room. I was speaking to the family and the patient about their upcoming treatment; you

came into the room and interrupted me. You reviewed the same information that I had already discussed with the family.

Next, connect them with the feeling that you had as a result of their action, i.e., "And after you did this, I was angry at you because you interrupted me, and I felt embarrassed and sorry for the family because they were receiving different messages."

Finally, articulate what you need the individual to do. Whenever you have a discussion with anyone, especially in a conflictual situation, it is very important to end the conversation with a request. You must tell people what you want them to do, i.e., "and what I would like you to do in the future is talk to me prior to interrupting me with the family when I am providing them with instructions. I believe it will help us get along better, and it will help the family not feel confused." Without this, it is difficult for the individual to correct his or her behavior in the future.

Here is what you do not want to say or do in this situation.

- Wait a long period of time to address the situation.
- Talk to others at work about how rude someone was to you.
- Hold the discussion in a public place.

For example, "You embarrassed me in front of a patient and his family last month. I've talked with others during the past few weeks, and they tell me you have done this before."

In this example, there were no "I" statements. The discussion took place far after the initial incident and in a public place. No facts were identified and, most importantly, no requests were made at the end of the conversation.

Lastly, the use of "you" produces a strong defensive response from others in a conversation. Take some time and think about conversations that you have had where someone used "you" instead of "I." How did that make you feel?

These guidelines may feel uncomfortable, but remember this: if you don't address conflictual situations, the anger you are experiencing will continue to grow. It is clear. To clarify this point, let me share with you a story from a nurse I met at one of my seminars.

Darlene was a 22-year-old new graduate who had just completed a 6-week job search. She chose to work in a local teaching hospital in Denver where she finished her nursing degree. She was extremely excited about the opportunity to further advance the skills that she learned in school at a hospital that was known for its educational programs, strong nursing leadership, and research opportunities. By most accounts, people would look at Darlene as an extremely beautiful young woman. She was about 5' 10" and had done some modeling during her college career. She was very aware of her looks and was convinced she wanted to be recognized for her intellectual abilities and her nursing skills.

When she entered the med/surge program, she was immediately placed with a senior nurse, Anita. Anita's role as a mentor was to provide formal orientation for Darlene for up to 6 weeks and ongoing mentorship through her first year. Anita had been a nurse for over 20 years. She was fairly new to this hospital, being employed for less than 3 years, but was highly recognized for her strong clinical skills and leadership abilities. Anita was a confident individual and was not shy about speaking out whenever she felt quality clinical care was being jeopardized. Most people described Anita as a bit overweight, quiet, and extremely professional.

The unit itself had over 25 nurses, the majority of them part-time individuals who had worked there for an average of 8 years. For the last 2 months they had been without a manager and had an interim manager, Shelly, from one of the adjacent units.

As the first 3 months passed, Darlene felt that she was achieving all of her goals. She felt confident in her skills and was feeling more and more independent each shift. Per hospital policy, a probationary evaluation was required at this point. The mentor was to complete a report and obtain feedback from other peers. Shelly asked to see Darlene to review her 3-month probation, which is standard practice. As she sat down to review it, Shelly started out with, "I have some bad news. I received some feedback from your mentor as well as other peers, and they are very concerned with your professionalism as well as your lack of progress in your clinical skills."

Darlene was stunned. She really didn't know what to say. She was shocked. She just continued to stare at Shelly with her mouth open. After a long pause, Shelly asked if she would you like her to read some of the comments, and she nodded in agreement.

"Your mentor stated that your attention to her instruction has not been consistent. She stated you appeared to be distracted by your peers and physicians as well as the family members. She stated that your punctuality and your attendance and energies seemed to be positive and moving in the right direction, but your commitment to learning clinical skills seems to be lacking."

Darlene sat back in her chair, looked at Shelly, and said, "I don't understand. All of my conversations with Anita have been positive. She has told everybody how wonderfully I am doing, and others have said that I am fitting in very well. If this isn't true, why didn't she just tell me?"

Shelly, looking a little puzzled, said that she had met with Anita and had been informed that Darlene had been given feedback throughout the 3 months. Darlene said, "That is not true. That has not occurred."

Shelly chose to move forward and review the corrective action plan. "What I need you to do right now is review this corrective action plan, agree with its direction, and sign it. You have to understand that you have another 3 months to turn this around, and I think you are able to do it." Still shocked, Darlene said to Shelly, "I'm already doing these things. I don't understand where this report came from." Shelly continued to encourage her to speak with Anita. She encourage her to sign the document and end the meeting.

Darlene signed the document and left the room. She was thankful that it was the end of her shift because she couldn't face anyone. Still shocked, she went home in tears. She had called her family looking for their advice about what to do. No one in her family told her to speak directly with Anita. Darlene had come to the conclusion that Anita just didn't like her and didn't want to work with her. She was so angry and hurt that she did not want to return the next day. She just wanted to quit.

I am sorry to say that Darlene never returned to work. She called Shelly, asked to rescind her signature on her probationary evaluation form, and told them she would be pursuing other opportunities.

Today, Darlene is a nursing professor. She shared this story with me after one of my seminars. She really loved what she was doing and found that the anger and the hurt from this specific experience stayed with her throughout her career. In fact, during her next 4 years in her job, she became very withdrawn. She avoided any public demonstration of her clinical skills. It was her way to protect herself. She said, "This was my first job out of school. I did not know how to deal with this type of stress or this kind of conflict. I didn't know where to turn or what to do."

I think it is important for us to remember, particularly with new graduates, that their coping strategies are minimal. Situations like this are not only detrimental to their career, they can affect their personal lives as well. Today Darlene is a confident woman, and she regularly practices the type of confrontation skills that I have outlined for you. She told me that what she learned from that initial experience was that the conflict that was present had little to do with her and more to do with Anita. She recognizes that Anita was very jealous of her skills, youth, and beauty, and she realizes that as a result, she felt threatened and out of control and she began acting out by sabotaging Darlene's career through this negative probationary evaluation.

Darlene told me she was more hurt by the lack of support from Shelly. If Shelly had brought the two parties together and addressed this conflictual issue, the outcome might have been different. Thank goodness Darlene stayed in the nursing profession and is teaching other young men and women the importance of not only the nursing skills but how to manage their stress and conflicts.

These last two truths provide you with an understanding of how to manage difficult personalities and conflict in your work world. The interventions I have shared with you are designed to create a positive outcome for you, your patients, and peers/supervisors. However, the stress that can be created is a concern. Stress can be detrimental to growth in your career and, potentially, to your health. The next truth will discuss burnout in health care providers and how to avoid it.

TRUTH #6:

AVOIDING BURNOUT IN YOUR JOB

Establish Boundaries to Protect Yourself

There is no revenge so complete as forgiveness.

—Josh Billings

Stress and Your Personality Style

We have covered how stress is prevalent in your work world, especially with regard to the last two truths in which we have reviewed staff and peer conflict. In today's world, I am extremely concerned about the potential for burnout in nurses and other health care employees. It goes without saying that the purpose of this book and the first five truths is to provide you with an opportunity *not* to perceive every situation as stressful, thus reducing your chance for burnout at work. Even with this in mind, burnout in the health care world is a real issue. I want to provide a further understanding of what it is and how you can avoid it.

Managing stress in our lives is a challenge for all of us. It is constant, but it can be managed very successfully. In a book by Valerie O'Hara, *Wellness 9 to 5: Managing Stress at Work*, she identified that "wellness at work is the active art of building resilience to job stress and daily life. It is more than the absence of illness. It is an approach to life. Wellness embraces the best of who we are in body, mind and spirit. It is proactive and preventative."

The previous truths aim to accomplish this. Wellness is the art of living life consciously and using the Control Reaction Map, along with the Success Steps model.

Some have encouraged me to devote an entire book (not just this one chapter) to discussing the psychological, physiologic, and spiritual effects stress has on our lives. For years you have read that different individuals perceive and process stress differently than others. O'Hara says that research has determined a correlation between specific behavior patterns and heart problems. Thus has been coined the term "Type A personality" for people with an urgent, aggressive, and hostile approach to life and the term "Type B personality" for those who are easygoing and relaxed. What is very encouraging is that she identifies that it is not so much the personality style that is more detrimental to your health but the individual's perception and management of stress. In other words, it's really how you interpret it and respond to what is going on. When we evaluate each personality style and understand exactly why people behave the way they do based on these personality styles, we better understand them. This can result in a response from you other than frustration, anger, and hostility—emotions which, over time, according to O'Hara, can lead to emotional issues as well as physiologic problems. O'Hara goes on to provide a number of tests to evaluate your work-related job stress, your resilience to stress, and your stress responses. I highly recommend this book so you can evaluate your specific stress issues even further to determine where you rank in her analysis.

To be fair to you, outside of evaluating O'Hara's stressor test, I think it is important for you to understand the initial signs of burnout and some precautions you can take. As we move into further truths and discuss difficult personalities and the development of a wonderful team, it is very important to have this understanding of burnout, along with the signs that might occur.

According to Katherine Kirkhart (1996) in an article titled "Caregiving and Burnout: Are You at Risk?" four stages of burnout can occur. The first stage is *idealistic enthusiasm*. This occurs when an individual enters a profession for the first time and feels very fresh and "over-committed" to having a positive impact.

The second stage is where *stagnation* sets in. Kirkhart goes on to state, "It becomes clear that the initial ideals do not contribute to workable goals and are likely to be unreachable." Multiple disappointments can occur, and the initial feelings of being in love with helping others no longer exist. The work seems to be unfulfilling where once it was exciting.

Stage three is when *frustration* occurs, "A type of relentless frustration that feels overwhelming. The frustration dilemma results from an awareness that the use of all available strategies, including working harder, are not bringing about the desired results. And, because time is limited, working harder is requiring repeated sacrifices." The frustration is a result of beginning to lose one's sense of self.

The final stage is *apathy*. This is when the work we do becomes mechanical and the feelings are subdued. The work that we do seems boring, and the people who we once loved seem distant from us.

Kirkhart also mentions compassion fatigue syndrome, and it is well worth mentioning here. Compassion fatigue syndrome involves feelings of sudden helplessness and confusion and most likely occurs as a result of a "helpers' secondary exposure to traumatic events when working with a victim." The person helping becomes traumatized, often marrying symptoms with those of the traumatized person, i.e., nightmares, fears and anxiety. As I discussed burnout with several nurses and health care workers, this syndrome presented itself on several occasions.

In "The Personality to Buffer Burnout," a 1998 article in *Nursing Management* by Mara Ponterdolph and Patricia Toscano, the authors evaluated critical care nurses who encountered stressful events daily to determine why some nurses were more "apt to buffer" such stressors and thus avoid the phenomenon known as burnout. They referred to many studies that have focused on burnout, particularly as it relates to specific types of nursing, and specifically the work of Christina Maslach. "The Maslach Burnout Inventory (MBI) was designed to measure certain aspects of burnout. It examines three subscales and identifies key aspects of the burnout syndrome: Emotional exhaustion, depersonalization and personal accomplishment. Maslach's framework proposes that burnout occurs, not because of the personality, but because of the negative environment." Ponterdolph and Toscano further state, "This is not a result of a one-time or acute care situation, but more of a chronic condition." Maslach further finds that the personality styles that are most likely to experience burnout are "unassertive, submissive, anxious, fearful and overburdened." Continuing, Maslach describes them as "impatient, intolerant and prone to act-out on angry impulses; they lack confidence and vision and a sense of personal accomplishment."

Reading this research from Maslach, I could not help but compare the 4-P Personality test with this research to identify who might be more prone to burnout. When I look at the personality characteristics "unassertive" and "submissive," I immediately think about the peacemakers. As I have stated before, I am very concerned about that personality style because they also appear to match other characteristics in the study, i.e., overburdened, fearful, and anxious.

However, when I look at the other personality characteristics identified, such as impatience, intolerance, and a tendency to act on angry impulses, I immediately think of the pointers and the processors. The point I would like to make is that the personality characteristics that they identified in this study support the characteristics of the 4-P Personality Style inventory.

In other research, Langemo (1990) studied the relationship between "personality hardiness, exercise activity, and work related stress." Her findings were these: "Higher exercise levels reported higher feelings of personal accomplishment. Personality hardiness was positively associated with personal accomplishment and negatively correlated with emotional exhaustion and depersonalization. Greater hardiness was linked to less work stress."

There is a lot of information here, so let's break it down. It seems logical that exercise, already identified as one of the top 10 ways to manage anger and conflict, is a mechanism that can make you feel better about yourself. Again, supporting the Success Steps theory, personality hardiness was positively associated with personal accomplishment. When you achieve, you feel better about yourself. We discussed that increased sense of self is accomplished through achievement, and this is another study that supports that statement.

What I did find was that personality hardiness was negatively correlated with emotional exhaustion and depersonalization, and greater hardiness was linked to less work stress. When you are exhausted and not connected to your peers or patients, you don't feel as good about yourself. You could also say that emotional exhaustion and depersonalization can lead you to feel out of control, and feeling out of control, again, gives you a lower sense of self.

Returning to the study by Ponterdolph and Toscano, they asked if the high levels of hardiness positively correlated with the low level levels of burnout in the critical care setting. I think for the purpose of understanding this study that we need to include their definition of burnout as well as their definition of hardiness.

Burnout: A syndrome of emotional exhaustion and cynicism that occurs frequently among individuals who do "people" work of some kind. As their emotional resources are depleted, workers feel they can no longer give of themselves at a psychological level. Another aspect is the development of negative, cynical attitudes about one's clients. A third aspect of the burnout syndrome is a tendency to evaluate one's self negatively, particularly with regard to one's work with clients.

Hardiness: A personality trait that moderates the effects of stress on health. People with hardy personalities have been shown to encounter less illness, despite the stressful situations they face, because they possess three adaptive characteristics: commitment, control, and challenge.

They concluded that the results of their study did not indicate that there was a relationship between personality hardiness and burnout. This finding supported Maslach's framework in which she felt the negative environment had more to do with burnout in the workplace than did the affected personality. It led them to focus more on the environment that they were working with and how the nurses perceived the environment. They closed the study with the focus that nurses could be taught how to manage high stress situations that occur daily. It is their (the nurses') perception that could be affected, causing a different understanding of stress and possibly avoiding burnout.

As we move to evaluate the 4-P Personality Styles and stress, it is important to point out these results. As Maslach's studies found, a negative environment can correlate with burnout in the workplace. However, the perception of what makes a negative environment is an area that can be affected. I am saying that nurses have the ability to create the type of "perceived" environment that they want. This takes training and development, but it can be accomplished.

Let's take some time and evaluate the relationship between the 4-P Personality Styles and stress and burnout.

> **The application of the first four truths will change your perception of what is a stressful situation.**

The Pointer

As pointers become stressed, they struggle with letting go of control. In fact, they become much more dominant toward others. They will increase delegation and become demanding (i.e., requesting frequent updates about patient care issues, projects, etc.). Others would describe pointers during these stressful times as hyperactive and intrusive, as evident in this quote from a nurse in Dallas describing her boss when she is stressed: "Why don't they just let me do my job and quit butting in?"

Here is an additional example of this style under stress from a nurse in Atlanta.

> John, a nursing supervisor, was always seen as a confident and strong leader. He was not much of a socializer but was very direct and to the point with his second shift staff. People liked him because of his decisiveness. Staff had noticed a difference, however, when the stress of the unit became high. They recalled one evening shift when the census was unusually high. There were repeated requests for additional beds, and staffing was short although there were staff in-house who were attending a mandatory training session. Staff found John stressed and noticed he began delegating beyond his normal routine. They found him taking over the charge nurse's role and identifying assignments and assessing each patient's acuity, determining if the patient was ready to move to another unit, a role that the staff nurse would normally perform. In addition, he began to be very curt in his responses to coworkers.

What is interesting about this case (as with any pointer) is that others can see this is occurring and how it relates to certain stressors.

Solutions

Pointers need to identify when they are out of their comfort zone. Once this occurs, they need to be specifically aware of their actions as they relate to this increased stress level. It is helpful to have somebody on their staff who understands how they respond to stress to help remind them if they become overactive and start to overdirect. It is also helpful for these personality styles to recognize these signs and remove themselves from the situation for a short period to regain their composure and enhance their leadership style.

Also, as a result of their increased directive behavior, pointers can become short with people, causing hurt feelings and anger among those individuals. There may be a need to repair any damage to relationships resulting from this behavior.

The Politician

We know the politician's focus is on innovative, creative, energetic, and brainstorming endeavors. The concern with this personality style is their lack of attention to detail and disconnection with their long-term projects.

As stress overtakes these personality styles, they increase their level of socialization. As a result, they become more scattered and lack consistency and structure. You can imagine what this does for staff. They become more frustrated themselves, and the chaos in their work world can increase. In addition to this, because of the stress, many politicians find themselves being more creative and energetic during this time, quite often identifying additional new projects to pursue. When this happens at the time when staff are in a stressful situation, this only adds to anger and resentment toward that individual. Let's look at an example of this style under stress as described by a nurse from Cincinnati.

Barb was a senior director of a pediatric program. She was hired because of her energetic personality style and her advanced clinical knowledge. During the past month, there had been several stressors that caused significant changes in her behavior. There were two accreditation reviews in a week, evaluations of a new clinical program, and end-of-quarter board meetings to review clinical and financial outcomes. Barb found herself increasingly staying later to prepare for all of these upcoming meetings and surveys. As a result of the stress, the staff started to receive additional emails. These emails were not only for updates of the survey and upcoming meetings, they also were additional projects that she announced for the first time to staff. She changed the usual monthly staff meeting to every week. Her agendas for the meeting also changed. They noticed her visibility increased, and she began telling everyone about these new projects, but she wasn't consistent. It just caused more confusion. The staff, already feeling pressure as a result of the surveys and the financial and quality review, felt even more stressed because of the additional ideas and projects Barb presented.

Solutions

Politicians will notice that during stressful times they have a higher sense of energy and excitement. They believe they have everything under control and view increased visibility as an opportunity to share additional ideas. As with pointers, it is helpful to have somebody who can inform the politicians that they are moving too fast and not being consistent with the staff.

The Processor

Let's look back at the processor. These are our most misunderstood individuals and they have a tendency to be our most dynamic leaders. We have learned that the processor's lack of interaction and reassurance to staff can sometimes be seen as being inattentive. Along with this, they have an incredible focus on processes as they relate to outcomes and attention to detail.

During times of extreme stress, you will find processors become more withdrawn from their employees. The amount of time that they interact and communicate with others lessens. You can imagine how this is perceived by others who already feel that their supervisor is unavailable to them. Along with this, their attention to detail becomes increased. They begin to micromanage a variety of different processes and become critical not of the outcomes but of the processes.

Here is an example as described by a nurse from San Jose.

Theresa is a director of a 26-bed cardiac unit. She has been employed for over 15 years at the same hospital and has steadily risen in her responsibilities to her current position. Initially, staff were taken back by her lack of enthusiasm and social ability, but they quickly realized her intelligence and commitment to fairness. During one stretch of the year, there were a number of resignations from her nursing staff, six in total. All were for legitimate reasons, but they still placed the unit and Theresa in a stressful predicament. As a result, other employees' shifts were changed to provide safe clinical supervision. Two travelers were hired, causing a significant increase in Theresa's budget. Theresa obviously became much more stressed. She demonstrated this through her increased management of the budget. She began sending detailed memos out reviewing all cost reports and asking staff to cut back in a variety of different areas. She became more isolated in her office, having less time to do initial rounds on the unit, and her interactions with her nursing staff were minimal. When she did rounds, she focused on patient care initiatives and was critical of her staff. This only confused the staff more.

Solutions

Processors need to be aware that stress causes them to become more isolative, more data driven, and more process oriented. They have to be aware of the results of this stress response on their staff, who often feel insecure and lacking in direction.

The Peacemaker

Referring back to the characteristics of the peacemakers, we know that their number one goal is to have a sense of peace and calmness among the team. They most assuredly are happiest when everyone else is content in their jobs. We also have learned that the weakness of a peacemaker is the inability to please everyone, and that level of frustration only grows with the size and complexity of the staff and program.

As peacemakers become stressed, they attempt to connect with all their employees. They project their level of anxiety to everyone. Through the constant interaction with others, they hope to assure that everyone has a sense of peace and comfort in the job. Problems can arise, as shown by this example from a nurse in Boston.

Johnail has been a nurse for 4 years and at this hospital for 2 years. Her first month on the job, Johnail quickly found out that she was in the middle of a constant battle among the staff nurses on the units, the emergency room, the practicing physicians, and the administration. She discovered that the decisions she had to make were extremely difficult and stressful, almost agonizing. No matter what she tried to do, somebody was not happy with her decision. If she moved the patient too quickly from the emergency room, the staff on the units were frustrated because they didn't feel that she supported them. When a patient was not placed in the right unit, the attending physicians were frustrated because the patient was not accessible. And, if additional staff were placed on the unit because of actual and/or perceived acuity, administration became frustrated with her. As these stresses increased, she attempted to meet with all these groups but to no avail.

Solution

Peacemakers succumb more easily to burnout. Other personality styles have the ability not to personalize the unhappiness of certain groups as much as the peacemakers do. Because of this, there never is any satisfaction in a peacemaker's job.

Peacemakers who continue to stay in nursing and other health care professions are not in supervisory roles but serve as staff. Why is it? It is simple: it's easier to belong to one group and please that group (or be asked to please that group) than it is to be a peacemaker and attempt (unsuccessfully) to please a multitude of groups.

See how easy it is for conflict to arise from some simple personality differences? We all approach life from a different perspective and style. As stress increases, all of us move to our dominant personality style, and this can cause conflict. This is a primary reason why health care work has become more demanding—not just because of the increase in the external stressors, but because of the impact of stress on the staff.

4-P PERSONALITY STYLE RESPONSES AND SOLUTIONS TO STRESSFUL BEHAVIORS

4-P Personality Style	Response to Stressful Behaviors	Management Solutions
Pointer	• Dominates • Delegates	• Give control • Don't micromanage
Politician	• Socializes and becomes scattered	• Limit project involvement • No new projects during this time
Peacemaker	• Seeks calmness • Solves problems	• Identify what is out of your control • Connect with staff • Review only the facts
Processor	• Isolative • Detail driven	• Be consistently visible to staff • Don't micromanage

Managing Burnout

So how do you avoid burnout? You are doing it now. Reconnecting to yourself, understanding who you are, and determining your Circle of Control are the steps to help you avoid and decrease the likelihood of burnout. The success you gain from this book will place you in a better position to avoid this situation and succeed in other areas.

One of the lessons you will learn is that there has to be a balance between your professional life and your personal life. As we speak about your specific self-worth, it will be much easier to understand how your actions in life need to balance and support who you believe you are.

It is also important not to lose objectivity. You must avoid over-identification with or personalization of patients or families. This loss of objectivity and separateness can cause an unhealthy role for the caregiver.

I want to return to truth five and revisit the top 10 guidelines for managing your anger and avoiding conflict. For your benefit, I have reprinted these below.

1. Acknowledge the moment that you are feeling angry and understand there is a source of this anger.
2. Return to your Circle of Control and evaluate the connection between your personality style and your specific self-worth as they relate to the conflict and anger.
3. Talk to someone in your external support system about the anger you are feeling. Do not keep this information inside. Determine the cause of your conflict.
4. Determine if the expectations regarding your conflict are realistic or unrealistic.
5. Identify the triggers to your conflict.
6. If the cause of the conflict is an individual at work, meet with that person to express your concerns. (Follow the conflict meeting guidelines in Truth #4.)
7. Evaluate your diet. Don't use excess food or alcohol to cope with the conflict.
8. Exercise regularly: walk, stretch, run. Get your blood flowing.
9. Meditate: find 15–20 minutes of down time to stop thinking and just be.
10. Leave work at work. It is not your home life.

We reviewed each of the 10 steps in detail in Truth #5, but there are a couple of points that I want to make as they relate to burnout. Based on all the research, the need to have a strong sense of self is an important indicator in avoiding stress and burnout. It is not a coincidence that the top 10 guidelines follow the outline of the Success Steps model by first helping you understand who you are through your Circle of Control.

I can't emphasize enough the need to review your Circle of Control throughout your career because it changes. The way many people find out it has changed is through stress and burnout. When they begin to identify the origin of their stress and their burnout, eventually it comes back to their Circle of Control. Although I do support the research that a negative environment dramatically affects one's stress level, the perception of what stress is is more important.

Let's look at some other suggestions on how to manage your life to reduce the possibility of increased stress and burnout. I want to spend some time referring to Valerie O'Hara's book, *Wellness 9 to 5: Managing Stress at Work*, especially in the areas of relaxation therapy and physical activity. I concentrate on this area because most of you are unaware of the immediate effects they can have, reducing your stress each day and minimizing the chance for burnout.

Let's begin by looking at O'Hara's recommendations for relaxation skills. The three areas she focuses on are conscious breathing, deep relaxation, and meditation.

Conscious Breathing

> *Healthy breathing techniques are easy to learn and can have profound effects on one's life.*
>
> —Menninger Clinic

Breathing helps us focus on the present. As we will review more in the next truth, stress and anxiety are a result of focusing on past or future issues. When we are in the "now" or the "being" aspect of our lives, there is no anxiety. Breathing helps us get there. O'Hara goes on to identify a specific exercise to explore your breathing patterns.

Step One
Sit with your eyes closed and begin with several slow, deep breaths. Relax your body, starting from your feet and moving towards your head. Take several minutes.

Step Two
Visualize an aspect of your life that causes you pleasure or happiness. This can be walking on the beach, talking to someone special, etc. For example, begin by visualizing your feet on the sand and in the water. Visualize the conversation you are having with that special person, what you are talking about, the smiles, and the smells in the air. You should do this for about 4 minutes, according to O'Hara, and then take a moment to step back and observe your breathing patterns. Have they changed? Do you feel more relaxed? Is there tension in your body?

Step Three
Now do the opposite and focus on a situation in your life that causes you tension, stress, or anxiety. Visualize this experience. O'Hara refers to visualizing being caught in traffic and the tension that arises from this. As you're visualizing, take a moment to assess your breathing. Has it changed? Do you feel tension anywhere else in your body? As you feel this tension, take a deep breath and release it.

Step Four
Reverse back to step two, to a visualization of something in your life that makes you feel calm. As you do this, notice the breathing change that occurs.

O'Hara points out that when people are stressed, they tend to constrict their chests, which can exacerbate the stress response. "By changing your breathing pattern, you can increase the flow of oxygen, balance the autonomic nervous system, cleanse the lymphatic system, maximize the exchange of carbon dioxide and oxygen, and decrease anxiety and tension." From personal experience, this breathing technique is very effective. It is a great way to immediately relieve stress at any time during the day.

Deep Relaxation

Deep relaxation goes beyond just breathing techniques and focuses on total relaxation of the muscles in the body. O'Hara describes how to use deep relaxation techniques. She says, "Focus your attention on each body part as indicated, and gradually tense, relax and observe the area. To tense an area, contract the muscles, gradually increasing the intensity to a full squeeze. The tensing allows you to then actively relax the muscles to a deeper at-rest level." She further states that this technique should take about 10 minutes to complete. The experience provides a deeper sense of relaxation by contrasting the tenseness with immediate relaxation. You can further enhance this experience by training yourself to focus specifically on that body part that is tensing and relax it.

I practice this on a regular basis each night, and it not only provides a sense of stress relief, but it also helps me get to sleep and have a better night's rest. This technique is more difficult to do at work, but it is a wonderful way to end the day.

Meditation

Meditation has picked up a great deal of acceptance over the last 5 to 10 years. What I have learned when I have spoken with nurses and other health care professionals is that they think they understand meditation, but they do not really know what it is. For one, meditation does take various forms. There are several types of meditation that O'Hara has identified, those being:

1. the quiet mind
2. quiet time
3. creative time
4. journaling

The *quiet mind* is by far the most discussed type of meditation. O'Hara identifies meditation as a "repeated practice of attempting to keep the attention on one designed object, thought or image. The meditator repeatedly focuses on an object without judging or criticizing the busy mind for wandering."

Meditation is not much more complicated than that, although the results can be extremely profound. The purpose of breathing techniques is to focus in on the present or the now; meditation is similar. Anxiety and stress result in focusing on the past or the future; meditation focuses on the present. O'Hara does identify four basic steps to having a successful "quiet mind" meditation.

1. A quiet environment. Any distraction can take you out of your focus on that specific object, thought, or image.
2. Find a comfortable sitting position.
3. Use some type of mental device to break any stressful thinking patterns, i.e., a word or a phrase.
4. Make sure you do not force any type of thought patterns in or out of your head.

She goes on to say that the techniques for quiet mind meditation begin with your natural breathing techniques and form a specific rhythm. She reminds you it is natural for your mind to wander during this process and not to become frustrated with that but just focus back on breathing to bring you to the center. After doing this for about 10 minutes, she recommends that you let go of the focus on breathing or a phrase and just be still and enjoy the inner quietness. As you practice this type of meditation, you will find that it is easier to settle into a breathing pattern and a state of inner peace.

Quiet time is described by O'Hara as "Attention in the present moment, whether it is being physically active or inactive." She describes further that an example of this would be a quiet walk, listening to the sounds of nature, gardening, hiking, reading, or watching the sunset. All of these exercises focus being in the "now" and on enjoying the surroundings.

Creative time focuses on revisiting or reinitiating hobbies and activities that you enjoy. It can be writing, singing, or any other activity. Again, the success of this meditation exercise is that it places you in the now.

Journaling is a different type of meditation but can be extremely effective for reducing stress and minimizing burnout. When I speak to processors, they prefer to do this type of meditation because it is something with which they are familiar. According to O'Hara, the purpose of journaling is to "give you the opportunity to clarify what is bothering you, so that you can look at healthier solutions." She further suggests a format when journaling your work-related entries.

1. Describe work stressors.
2. Identify feelings and perceptions.
3. Identify healthy options to manage that stress.

All four of these meditation techniques are very helpful. I cannot emphasize enough to you the importance of using these tools. Some are more difficult to use at work, but at least one (breathing exercises) can be done anywhere at any time.

Physical Activity

Until I started writing this book, my physical activity level had been very high. I have noticed in the last year that, as a result of my busier schedule from my seminars and writing, that I have made less time for this. I can tell you that I feel a great deal of difference in my emotional and stress levels. Without my regular exercise, I feel less productive, grumpier at times, and not as optimistic. I am sure lack of exercise and physical activity affects others in a variety of different ways. This is how I respond.

Because I am talking to nurses and other health care professionals, I do not believe it is necessary in this book to tell you that one of the leading causes of death in the United States is heart attacks, followed by cancer, strokes, and other blood vessel diseases. I know you understand this and the importance of exercise. What I am going to provide for you is my list for creating a successful and realistic program.

1. Write down what it is you like to do for exercise. Please don't put down what you think others want to hear or what you've read. I want you do identify what you enjoy doing. I don't care if it's throwing a Frisbee, playing with your kids at a local pool, or taking a walk every night with your dog. Just put down what you like. This will be extremely important.
   A.
   B.
   C.
2. Schedule a time in which you can do this activity or a combination of these activities at least three times a week for 30 minutes.
3. Create a schedule and monitor the progression of these exercises by creating a check list and marking appropriately as you accomplish it.

I am not making this complicated, and I'll tell you why. You can find over 200 exercise books in the stores, on the Internet, and on television that will give you all types of advice on what to do, and I encourage you to find something that will fit your lifestyle. I'm more concerned that you get started and that you connect some sense of enjoyment with what you are doing. If you don't, you will not do it. You know this, and I know this because you have gone through this cycle before.

All I am saying is begin to move and move in a way that you enjoy. Monitor this and reward yourself for your success.

Nutrition

O'Hara has a wonderful quote in her book, which is from Covert Bailey, *Fit or Fat*: "If you can lube your car with it, don't eat it." I could not agree more. Here are my top three nutritional habits to adopt.

Document what you are eating. For a stretch of 3 days, write down everything you eat. Understand what you are and are not putting in your body.

Is there is any relationship between stress in your life and your eating habits? When you are evaluating what you have eaten for the last 3 days, start to look at the stress that is occurring and if there is a correlation with the type of food you are eating.

Create a plan to reduce the number of calories in your diet (assuming from your review of your food intake that you would like to alter this).

I hope this truth has helped you understand the signs and symptoms of burnout so that you can avoid it. I have seen too many nurses and other health care professionals experience burnout. I am extremely concerned that this could happen to you. Please be aware of the signs, and follow the first five truths.

TRUTH #7:

CREATING GREAT TEAMS AND GREAT MANAGERS

It Doesn't Just Happen;
It's Hard Work and
It Can Happen for Your Team.

Vision comes alive when everyone sees where his or her contribution makes a difference.

—Unknown Author

Congratulations! You have made it through the first six truths, and you have a better sense of who you are and who you want to be. You have the tools to create a peaceful and productive environment, and, more importantly, you have a better sense of confidence because you have the tools to interact successfully with families for whom you care and the staff with whom you work.

Our work would not be complete, however, if we did not talk about how we help develop our peers (improving their clinical skills while connecting them with the team), how we get along with each other and create a productive and healthy team. I do not have to tell you the difficulties of having to work with so many different types of personalities. You have experienced that firsthand. In this chapter, I will share with you some wonderful stories about nurses and their struggles to connect with their work. We are going to evaluate the use of Success Steps tools in conjunction with the most up-to-date management strategies to create a productive work world for you.

During my interviews with nurses and other health care personnel I found that they generally do not believe that the work world they want is even a possibility. They believe that chaos is present in every health care organization and that there is a disconnect among managers, directors, and staff. This has been their consistent experience. More importantly, they feel they have little or no ability to affect or change the system, and, of course, when you believe you can do nothing to change your experience, you will not even try. On the other hand, those who have read this book or attended my training seminars do have the tools to create a different environment for themselves and the team. As they begin to apply these tools, they find their beliefs—and their experience—changing. They are proof that you can create an environment that changes your culture and becomes a model for other organizations to emulate.

Why is it important to develop the team? The answer, quite simply, is that there are things that you as an individual cannot accomplish alone without the team. The influence of many has a much stronger impact on change than the influence of one person working alone. Again, you may think developing a strong team is not possible, but, in fact, it is. Not only will I teach you how to create a culture that is wonderful, but you are also going to learn how to mentor staff to fit into this culture and train your managers to become the managers you want them to be. The results of all this are simply dynamic. Let's get started!

You now have all the tools to make this happen. Let's refer to the Success Steps model to understand exactly what needs to be done first.

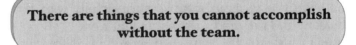

There are things that you cannot accomplish without the team.

In the third truth you learned that the first step of the Success Steps model is to initiate and develop trust. When working with a team, this is also true. Your goal is to create a sense of control for the entire team. Once this occurs, the team can communicate with respect.

There can be many obstacles to accomplishing this goal. At times it can seem nearly impossible to get everyone on the same page. It only takes one co-worker, one doctor, one technician, or one manager to remove the trust from the team and keep everyone functioning on step one. You know what I am saying. You have experienced this. With

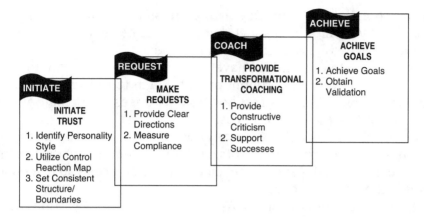

The Success Steps Model to Emotional Connection

this negativity in the air, co-workers begin talking about each other, cliques form, and managers may play favorites. You cannot survive long in this world. Those that do have created an experience devoid of joy, teamwork, and support. This atmosphere attracts similar employees and discourages those interested in a productive, healthy environment. Just look at the story of Becky from the second truth. Becky would have continued to survive in her work world; she would have remained there as an angry person or left as a bitter one.

I can't tell you how many teams I have evaluated and found on step one. I am not talking about new programs that have opened; I am talking about programs that have been in existence for a number of years with staff that have been there just as long. They have never experienced any other level for a team. Maybe you can relate to this. Maybe your team has never grown beyond the trust stage.

What I am pleased to tell you is I have seen organizations that have been beyond the trust step. Many have made it to Step Four, and some are continuing to move past Step One. It can be done. The experience can be amazing, and if you think that it can't happen to you, you are wrong.

Success Steps

Initiate Trust

We have identified personality styles and the importance of understanding your peers' personality styles. This is an area that causes teams to remain on Step One. Not understanding the various personality styles and the distinct characteristics of each one can result in continuous conflict among team members.

Refer back to the stories I have shared with you. Evaluate the relationships in your department or unit. Begin to recognize the different personality styles and how conflict arises as a result of not understanding these differences.

Learn and revisit the Control Reaction Map. Identify how you relate to your peers, supervisors, and other members of the health care team, and ask yourself if each interaction places you in a position to feel in or out of control.

Look at your relationships. Assessing the Control Reaction Map, in what direction have these relationships gone? You do not have to experience the same results.

Finally, let's look at structure and boundaries. There is a common denominator in all the organizations who remain on Step One. The rules, the regulations, the policies and procedures, and the communication patterns are all inconsistent. The purpose of having consistent structure and boundaries in an organization is not to control you or your peers or the team. The purpose, very clearly, is to put you in a position to succeed, to direct all of your energies in a productive direction.

How many of you experience inconsistencies each day in your job? This can be how your schedule is completed, how patients are admitted and discharged, what benefits certain staff receive compared to management, or disciplinary action. The list can go on forever, and if you don't believe that these inconsistencies prevent you from experiencing a different work world, then you are mistaken.

> **Organizations that remain on Step One lack structure and boundaries.**

We stated at the beginning of this book that we would not focus on your external conditions, just your perceptions. However, it is appropriate to discuss these external conditions in the context of having consistent structure and boundaries. If you do not put yourself or your team in a position to succeed, it will be more difficult for you to manage your external world.

So what do you do? This is a management and a team decision. The first step is for the group to agree that there should be a set of consistent rules for everyone. Start simple: start with everybody arriving at work on time, or agree to a certain level of respect for each other, how you will treat each other, and how you will not. (Showing up on time is a demonstration of respect.)

One hospital I consulted with decided after the seminar that they were going to begin the process of developing structure and boundaries among their team by creating a guideline on how to respect each other, families, and anybody who walked on the unit. It took 6 weeks to get their team together and to feel comfortable enough to be able to identify, document, and collectively sign what they believed was a fair and appropriate respect guideline. They attempted to bring in a variety of disciplines to support this effort, and this was not successful.

With the approval of their manager, the vice president of patient services, they posted these guidelines throughout their unit. Within 3 weeks, the guidelines were taken down. You may ask why. One of the guidelines stated that everyone was to be treated in a respectful and kind manner. An interaction occurred on that unit where this was not demonstrated. The entire team agreed that if a rule was not followed, the team would confront the individual or individuals to redirect them. This did not occur. The team became frustrated, feelings were hurt, and the guidelines were discontinued.

I share this with you because it is an important point. Developing trust in Step One takes a commitment from everyone, and you have to understand developing trust means that you will support the principles that the team has identified at all times. The satisfaction of experiencing a team on Step Three and soon to be on Step Four is amazing, so amazing that it is worth going through these growing pains to create a trusting environment.

There is a positive twist to this story. Six weeks later, the team did get back together. I was able to intervene with that group, and they were able to process and realign themselves with the initial principles. The guidelines were reinstated and posted.

This is a great deal of work. Being in the culture of a group to prepare them to move past Step One is a full-time job, and it is not just for a manager, it's for the entire team. If the team doesn't decide to move past Step One, the greatest manager in the world won't be able to help.

Make Requests

So what does this team look like when they move on to Step Two? Because boundaries and structures are in place, the team is able to be productive, following directions and making requests of other individuals. This is very new for many people. They have described this step by saying, "It really feels like we know what we are doing here" or "The program really looks good. We seem to be functioning well together."

For some, this is the first experience of not having a unit in ongoing and daily conflict. It could be their first experience of having limited gossip and backstabbing by staff members. One nurse I spoke with said, "It's like trying on a new dress and making it fit. You think it looks good, but you are not sure if you are really comfortable yet." The one thing that it does tell you is you have truly made it past Step One. You know this because requests are being followed. Teams that continually choose not to follow requests and directions are teams that are still struggling to develop a sense of trust among themselves.

Provide Transformational Coaching

If you walk into any bookstore and go to the management section, you could probably spend a full year reading all the books on how to manage people and coaching. What has to be in place for someone to be coached? Based on the Success Steps model we know that there has to be trust and they have to have a sense of pride in what they are doing. They also have to want to be coached. Not everyone does; not everyone knows how. What prevents most people from not being coached is the fact that they don't feel very good about themselves. As a result, they protect themselves and become defensive. For some, moving along the Success Steps model is much more difficult than it is for others. Why? There are many factors, including their own growth and development issues, relationship issues, and past experiences. The good news is that everyone *can* be coached. It is a matter of trying to find the right formula to get people to trust you, to follow your requests, and then to lower their defenses so they will allow you to coach them.

Coaching is not solely a management function. Coaching is a team function. In fact, coaching is much more effective when members of the team decide to support each other. Refer back to Truth #5 when we spoke about conflict among peers. Look at some of the causes of those conflictual situations. One area we discussed was envy. It is difficult to coach somebody who is continually jealous of others. This is something that can be difficult to manage, but it is possible. It is also possible to alleviate a lot of that envious, jealous behavior just by having the individuals sit down and discuss the issue. How many people with whom you work do you truly feel comfortable offering criticism to? I have met very few health care workers who ever address with their peers ways to improve for fear of being per- ceived as a know-it-all, bossy, or just rude. However, I'll tell you this; until the team can begin to develop each other, you will never arrive at Step Four on the Success Steps model, and I would even argue that you have not made it past Step One as a result of the inability to develop each other.

Achieve Goals

When you achieve goals, you celebrate. Look at your organiza- tion, your program, and your staff. Do you celebrate? Celebration doesn't mean it always has to be a work function. Celebration can mean getting together with people to appreciate the accom- plishment that you have made and your support of each other. These are usually the events that the politician's personality style organizes.

What I am *not* saying is to go out with your peers to complain about management or to complain about a variety of different sce- narios. This is not celebrating. Negative socialization is a result of feeling out of control and is not the same as positive socialization, celebrating achievement.

The other aspect of achievement is validation. Validation is the occurrence of introspection between two or more individuals. Usually, it is staff who have acted inappropriately at some point in their professional relationship(s), maybe because they were defen- sive and protecting themselves, but during the achievement step, the staff took the opportunity to possibly thank the individual for continuing to work with them and apologize for their behavior. This does not happen often, but when it does, it can be one of the most rewarding experiences.

Team Development Strategies

I want to take this opportunity to provide you with a more concrete, step-by-step process for developing your team. Below are the top 10 team development strategies. Please review these. I will discuss each one in detail.

1. Clearly identify your mission statement.
2. Post the mission statement on your unit/program.
3. Develop and post "Respect Guidelines" that support the mission.
4. Identify the management philosophy (decentralized).
5. Identify the organizational structure, along with short- and long-term strategies.
6. Initiate "15 minutes of fame" with all staff members (the time to review the mission, values, and strategic initiatives).
7. Develop an operationalized communication plan for both information sharing and problem solving.
8. Create a staff participatory committee structure.
9. Celebrate achievements from strategic initiatives.
10. Develop an active and ongoing staff recognition program.

First, you need to begin by clearly articulating the mission and values statement. Everything, and I mean everything, will be a direct result of your mission and values statement and how they are acted on by you and your staff. For example, if you are the leader in improving child health throughout the country, how you embark on this will affect the results you achieve. If you are teaching staff about collaborative work methods but do not reflect that in your overall mission, your staff will get a mixed message. They, in turn, will be unclear in their communications with other staff and patients, creating even more confusion.

However, it does not stop there. How do you take your mission statement and operationalize it to your unit? And, how do you get everyone to agree with this strategy?

This can be very difficult because getting the entire team, not just nursing but also physician services and other disciplines, to have the same direction is a difficult task. That is why you must be very clear about your mission statement and how you will demonstrate your mission on your unit or in your program.

Next, after you have identified your mission statement, you need to post this throughout your organization or unit, have all staff review it and sign that they understand it. Again, this needs to be operationalized so everyone understands what it means in their day-to-day work, and you must model this for them.

Third, there has to be an agreement about respectful behavior. Everyone must respect one other. Sounds easy, but every day there are many acts of disrespect that erode the foundation of a unit and its trust. To ensure this respectful environment exists, some hospitals have created a "respect guideline" that they post on their unit for all staff and families to see. Understand that you just cannot post this and all will be well. Creating and making the guideline visible is just the beginning of the cultural shift. An internal marketing plan needs to be developed to inform everyone what is happening and why this is important. All staff must support this. The real test will come when someone demonstrates behavior not in support of the guideline. How this behavior is addressed will be the real signal about the mission and values statements. This is a great beginning and creates a foundation for success on step one.

Next, managers must be aware of communication styles. They must ensure that their staff understands how information is shared in the organization and on the unit and that it is acted on consistently. Staff must have a clear understanding of how decisions are made. For example, your staff needs to know if you believe in a decentralized management style or an autocratic one. They need to know how you make decisions: do you plan to make the majority of your decisions on your own and inform your staff of them, or do you include your staff in the decision-making process? Again, without knowing the overall management structure of your team, the team members are not sure how to succeed. They struggle with this because they do not know how to interact in a nondescript management structure. This confusion creates a sense of loss of control. A complete plan must be created that provides a clear structure and boundaries for the staff. It is imperative that this is clear to the staff and that you are consistent in implementing this plan.

Why is this so essential? Clear structure and an understanding of what to expect and how to operate provide a sense of control to staff. In the absence of this, they spend their energy creating their own rules. This keeps them in a constant state of doubt and feeling out of control. You all have experienced organizations like this. You feel safe with a manager who has his or her act together and is fair to everyone (consistent).

What about all those different management styles? Let's choose the style that is going to support the use of the Success Steps model. Participating management (decentralized management) provides staff with the best opportunity to be in control. It is a style that encourages staff to be in control of their work environment and, subsequently, their outcomes.

If it is that good, why don't more managers adopt this style? Many managers do not use it because they feel very uncomfortable giving control over to the team. Remember the Circle of Control, the package each manager brings to the team, and the Control Reaction Map. If managers feel out of control, they will be less likely to give away control to the staff.

Up to this point, we have put the skeleton on the team. We've outlined exactly who is a part of this team and specifically how they relate to each other and the rules and values that will be governing them. Now is the time to ensure that everybody is on the same page. Everybody must affirm the mission, the communication structure, and management philosophy. To accomplish this I encourage the use of the "15-minute meeting." This is a meeting between the manager and each individual staff member. In actuality, it's about 30 minutes, but the idea is that every staff member meets with his or her direct supervisors for a brief period to discuss the structure of the program. This is essential.

In each of my director positions I have implemented this strategy. It accomplishes two things. It provides staff members an opportunity to understand what is expected of them, and it helps them get to know you as the director. When you have completed the meetings with each staff member, there are three statements that I encourage you to place in front of your staff. Their task is to choose the one statement that most accurately reflects their current mindset regarding your plans. The three statements are:

1. I understand exactly what you are asking from me and what the structure of the team will look like. I love it, and I want to do it.
2. I know exactly what you are asking of me and what the structure of the team will look like, and I don't know how to do it. Would you teach me?
3. I know exactly what you are asking of me and what the structure of the team will look like. It doesn't fit my style, and I don't think I can work here.

You are going to find that not all of your employees will select the first or second statements and will, instead, choose the third one.

This can be very healthy; it gives you the opportunity to assist them in finding another job, helping them leave an organization they feel they will be unable to work in, and, as a result, experience a sense of empowerment.

Please do not get me wrong. I don't mean to sound too simple or even cold. It is quite appropriate to ask further questions and ensure employees understand exactly what kind of structure you are setting up, but you also have to respect that they do understand what you have communicated very clearly and have made a conscious decision that this is not for them.

On the other hand, you will also find individuals who have selected responses one and two, but during the implementation phase of your team's programs, you discover that their actions do not match their verbal support of the program. This is a key time for the manager and the team. As the manager, you must sit down face to face with anybody who is demonstrating behavior that is not in support of the structure of the team. This isn't easy, but it can be very effective and ensures the stability of the team structure. Not only are you supporting your entire team by doing this, you are, ultimately, supporting individuals in their own work experience.

We spoke earlier of the value of a clear communication plan for both information sharing and problem solving. You will excel in this area if you can create a committee structure to aid in managing issues related to patient care and the work world. The more staff can participate in these decisions, the more they will feel in control, and the more likely you can progress through the success steps. In a decentralized management structure, staff not only need to be a part of identifying problems, they need to be active in finding solutions to achieve the identified outcomes. Nothing is worse for staff and for the team than developing a system that allows them to identify problems and solutions only to have them not be supported or implemented. This will quickly decrease their resolve in supporting this kind of atmosphere.

The next part that is very important is to celebrate achievements with all of your accomplishments and outcomes. Finally, you want to develop an active and ongoing staff recognition program. This is extremely important because it recognizes those individuals who support the philosophy of the team and assures the team that there will be rewards for demonstrating this type of behavior.

In truth, this chapter could be neverending. The amount of information for staff and managers is endless. It seems there is a new book or magazine article each week telling you how to manage, communicate, or deal with conflict. Although many of these re-sources are good, it is very easy to get overwhelmed. Here is what I want you to remember: keep it simple! Be fair and consistent and really know your staff. The hope I have for all administrators is that you will be able to use the Success Steps model in everyday man-agement decisions. It is simple enough to memorize and guide all your interventions and interactions. Good luck!

Developing Managers

Let's focus our attention on managers. The role of manager has become the most difficult position in today's health care world. At the same time, it is the most important role in the success of an or-ganization. I believe most of you who have been in a managerial role understand this dichotomy. You are placed between the front-line staff and upper management. Trying to please both entities can seem impossible. As our environment becomes more complex and staff replacements become increasingly costly, a sophisticated skill set is required that currently doesn't exist. This skill set must include strategies to guide the manager in implementing the hospital strategies, managing patient and family complaints, and ensuring staff are satisfied and retained. If this does not occur, managers can be a cause of the dysfunction of the unit.

How do we deal with and prevent this dysfunction?

First, you have to understand how managers can contribute to this dysfunctional workplace. Many managers feel uncomfortable with their own emotions and attempt to skip Step One, going straight to Step Two (Make Requests). They are much more comfortable direct-ing, implementing policies and procedures, and tell staff what to do. What they fail to recognize is that when the team does not follow the directions provided in the policies, it actually sets up a self-perpetu-ating loop. The team doesn't follow directions, so the manager contin-ues to push the policies and procedures rather than going back to Step One (Trust), resulting in an even greater lack of trust from the team and more frustration on the part of the manager. This is a serious discon-nect. They are missing this key strategy for developing a successful team. In reality, the majority of a manger's time needs to be spent on gaining trust or ensuring that trust continues and is not eroded.

This may seem obvious as it's being described here, but why don't many managers realize this? Return to the Control Reaction Map.

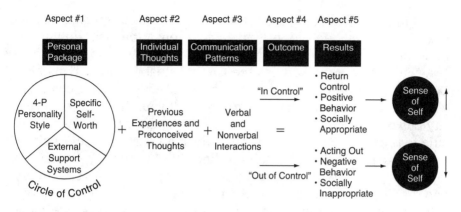

The Control Reaction Map

As a result of managers not having the skills or training to manage people, they find themselves feeling out of control. When this occurs, they act out or try to protect themselves by attempting to control others through the use of policies and procedures. They see this approach as a way to regain control. Obviously it doesn't work, and their staff begin to feel out of control and react as well, and then everyone is back to needing step one.

In a 2000 publication from the Nursing Executive Center, *Reversing the Flight of Talent: Executive Briefing*, three major strategic directions were identified to retain nurses.

1. Strengthen new hire support systems.
2. Address the top three drivers of nursing departure.
3. Develop front-line Chief Retention Officers.

The success of these strategies begins with the development of trust among the entire team. Without this, these and other strategies would not be possible.

The first strategy, strengthening new hire support systems, focuses on the high turnover rate for new hires. The research shows this higher turnover rate is a result of poor training and support systems in the first year of a new nurse's tenure. Think about this: being adequately trained and having support systems or mentors provides you with the ability to feel in control and eventually begin developing a higher sense of self. When these two do not exist, turnover rate increases. Or, stated another way, when you do not successfully achieve Step One (Trust), you are unable to achieve your goals.

Strategy two addresses the top three drivers of nursing departure. They have been identified as compensation, scheduling options, and intensity of work.

Again, these areas address the Control Reaction Map dynamics. Being compensated demonstrates a sense of worth. Having control of your schedule allows you to be in control of your life, and the intensity of work, as outlined in the first truth, equates to nurses feeling able to provide quality patient care, which reflects a sense of self.

Strategy three, developing front-line Chief Retention Officers, is most likely the top strategy for supporting the Success Steps theory and the Control Reaction Map. As in strategy one, having a relationship with your supervisor and other senior staff is the single most important reason why staff members stay and develop in their roles. To illustrate this, let's look at a story of a new graduate and how a lack of training and support affected her career.

Diane had just completed her nursing degree from a local junior college. She had spent the last 2 years working as a mental health aid in a community psychiatric program. Diane appeared comfortable as a nurse because she knew the program and the staff. She told me she felt confident making the transition.

Diane was well liked by all because of her warm personality and her energy at work. She didn't anticipate anything changing as she changed roles. Staffing at this small community hospital was much like any other hospital its size. Diane quickly found herself with an orientation that lasted less than a full week. Soon after this, she was placed in charge several evenings a week.

During my interview with her, she reflected back to this time and told me, "It wasn't the short orientation or the early charge assignments that stressed me the most; it was the fact that there was little support from other nurses or management. They all just expected me to figure it out. Sure, they asked me how I was doing, but they did not really appear to care what my response was. It felt like my peers were tired, burned out, just wanted me to do my job and not burden them. My director just wanted the shift covered. Maybe they felt differently, but that's what it seemed like."

Within 2 months, she was asked to take charge of the evening shift on a permanent basis. She was flattered they had asked her. She had reservations but ignored them and accepted the position. She soon believed she should have listened to those reservations.

Within the first week she began to feel unprepared. She had never completed schedules but was put in a position to post her first one with several requests from her staff regarding time off.

Once the schedule came out, she was inundated with complaints. She was overwhelmed. She immediately went to her director, who was supportive but was unable to improve the situation. Issues like this only got worse. There were staff conflicts, accusations that she was playing favorites, and long hours.

Diane couldn't take it any longer. One early evening shortly after her shift began, the unit became loud and two patients began arguing. Two of Diane's staff began to intervene. In the process, the argument became more heated. Her staff were struggling, and Diane didn't know how to help. Later, she told me she had never felt more useless in her career than at that moment. One of the patients pushed the other one, causing him to fall into a staff member. Both hit the wall and fell to the ground. Staff subdued the other patient, but the damage was done.

This staff member's head had hit the wall, causing a large laceration and a temporary loss of consciousness. The patient on the floor quickly tended to her. He looked up at Diane and asked, "Can't you keep us safe?" Diane just stood there. She knew he was right. In fact, she knew all of her staff were thinking the same thing.

After treating the staff member and sending her to the ER, Diane walked to the director's office. She did not knock. She rushed in and yelled, "I can't take it anymore!" She was crying and shaking. The director responded by asking what was wrong, but even he knew it could not be solved in a conversation. She grew even angrier saying, "What's wrong? Everything!" And with that, she took her keys, threw them on the ground, and told the director she quit. She turned, ran out of the office, and never returned.

The reason I am sharing this story with you is that I was the director. I was the one who failed to provide training, support, and mentoring to a new nurse who did not have the leadership (clinical) skills for this type of position. However, I ignored that and assumed she would just figure it out and learn as she went.

Later, I had a chance to see Diane to talk about this experience. She was quite gracious and agreed she had not been prepared for the role. She left nursing and started her own business. She agreed to let me share this story in the hope that it would help other managers and new staff.

It is quite easy to see the mistakes I made. I quickly eroded the trust I had with Diane. She was regularly demonstrating her feeling of being out of control, but I did not respond adequately. Yes, I was supportive, but not to the point that Diane was feeling in control. Instead, I kept giving her requests (Step Two), and this did not work.

There is further research to support that building trust is the first and most important step in developing the team. As you can see from the previous story, the quality of the emotional connection that staff members make with their peers, as well as managers and supervisors, is and will continue to be the single most important reason nurses and other health care personnel stay in or leave their current positions. The first step in developing trust begins with this relationship. From there, we can begin to further develop each team member and the entire team.

As managers continue to grow and develop, they learn a valuable lesson. They begin to have a deeper understanding of themselves. As many have stated to me, they don't have a choice but to learn about themselves. As we evaluate the remaining areas of the Control Reaction Map, managers' awareness of their specific self-esteem issues is crucial. To know yourself, you have had to identify your specific self-worth list and ensure that your energies match the sequential characteristic order.

Without the conscious understanding of their Circles of Control, managers have identified that they have limited success in their role. What about your 4-P Personality Style? It goes without saying that you have to have an understanding of your style and the pros and cons of that style as a manager. Throughout this book, we have reviewed the various 4-P Personality Styles and evaluated their strengths and weaknesses. Below is a review of these styles as it relates to being a manager.

Processor. We know that the processor is a sequential thinker and very independent. Managers with this style usually are very organized. They believe in a clear structure and support a communication structure the follows a chain of command. They pride themselves on having a well-run program.

The concerns they bring to the team are that they tend to be logical thinkers and struggle with the idea of developing trust with their employees. It is not that they are incapable of this; they have a difficult time letting go of control and may limit their interaction with others. They struggle with staff who do not quickly understand their system. They need to surround themselves with people who help them understand their staff and who support a participatory program.

Politician. Politicians bring energy and enthusiasm to the management role. Their ability to unite the team and create a sense of purpose is second to none. They have the ability to work with other departments and outside systems effectively.

The concerns or pitfalls for politicians are their high rate of speed and lack of consistency. They have a tendency to move quickly without a clear plan or direction and will not always keep the staff apprised of their direction when they do have one. They are not detailed individuals and tend to look at only the big picture. When you are implementing a plan and the details are lost, staff can feel lost as well. This can make the team feel left behind or not understanding how to achieve goals. Politicians can also lose interest in a project, quickly moving to another one. They may also forget to give their staff credit or let others have the spotlight. To be successful, they must surround themselves with individuals who can help them slow down and develop a comprehensive plan.

Pointer. Pointers are natural at taking the lead and being in charge. They can multitask and delegate effectively and they are well respected by their staff because of these traits. They also provide a sense of security because of their presence and confidence.

The directive style of pointers, however, can make others feel that they have little input. This style can appear controlling, minimizing staff participation and fostering a dependent group. The problem with this is when the pointer is not present, the operations stall. Pointers need to surround themselves with people who can ensure that decisions are made collectively at times and that staff have clear participation. The other thing that pointers need to do is be aware that they may not be as visible as they need to be. Because they are so busy multi-tasking, they may not make themselves visible consistently.

Peacemakers. Peacemakers are wonderful at creating a sense of team. They are sensitive and caring to their staff. They are well liked. Their motivation is to provide a sense of safety and support, and they work diligently to accomplish this. They encourage and foster team decision making and are usually not defensive, making them easy to approach.

The concern with the peacemaker style is their inability at times to make decisions. This stems from their avoidance of conflict. It is this avoidance that can cause a staff to feel a lack of leadership and direction. Because they avoid conflict, they may not be able to redirect staff who demonstrate inappropriate behaviors. They need to surround themselves with people who can communicate a clear and direct message and correct any confusion or conflict.

Providing a sense of structure and consistency in your organization will help staff be successful. You need to understand this. Structure and boundaries allow people to decide what they can and cannot do and the consequences of those decisions. This is empowering. If they understand what is expected of them, they have a better chance to feel in control, to succeed and feel better about themselves. Without consistency, staff do not understand what is expected of them, and they feel less in control, taking them down that road of the Control Reaction Map.

Let's move on to Step Two of the Success Steps model. The majority of managers that I have interacted with feel much more comfortable moving into a management position and beginning on Step Two, only to find they are not reaching desired goals. It appears easy to focus on policies, procedures, and directing others. It is clear that managers quickly find that staff do not comply with their requests because trust has not been developed.

Why is it that managers have a fear of initiating trust? It is because they do not have a sense of themselves or an understanding of their Circle of Control. When the managers do not have an understanding of themselves, it is very difficult for them to spend their energy on Step One. These individuals quickly move to Step Two. In the case of Becky, the manager made a feeble attempt at initiating trust but quickly moved to Step Two, Make Requests. I want you to understand this concept because this is the number one management mistake that is made.

Step Three, Coach, is one of the most rewarding steps, as I have stated before. It is a shame that many managers do not experience this step because of the avoidance of initiated trust.

As a manager, it is important to remember, that coaching is not just providing feedback. It is a give-and-take relationship between the manager and the employee. It is important for managers to allow employees to provide feedback about them and their performance. If managers are not comfortable with themselves, this can be a very difficult task.

The last step, which is achieving your goals, is an area of great concern in the health care environment (specifically in nursing). Nurses have a hard time at acknowledging their accomplishments and celebrating their achievements. As a manager, you need to create the culture of celebrating your successes. Organizations that never make it to Step Four and survive day to day on Step One do not understand how to celebrate their achievements. As a manager who understands this process, you can change that.

You will also note that at this step validation will occur. (We discussed this earlier in this truth.) It is a time as a manager when all of your work with staff members and even patients and families will be validated. This means individuals will approach you and acknowledge that their behavior or their actions may have not been desirable. In some cases, they may even apologize and thank you for sticking with them through the tough times.

This is what makes the Success Steps model for managers extremely valuable. It provides a systematic strategy for creating a work environment that develops people. In addition to this, it provides a retention program. After one of my seminars, a nurse approached me and commented that the Success Steps model reminds her of bronco bull riding. Puzzled, I asked her to elaborate on her comparison. She said, "Your goal is to ride the bronco for a period of time. You start by getting on and secure yourself and holding on for the entire 60 seconds. At times, you think you are in control and moving in the right direction and in a moment, you can be out of control." I thought the analogy was very appropriate, and it helped me better understand how staff and managers perceive the Success Steps. I wanted to share that with you.

I want to also take this opportunity to look at some other popular management techniques that support the Success Steps model. There are many popular business and management books out there to provide guidance for you on how to develop a team. Ken Blanchard, the author of numerous books, has provided a great deal of research and direction in this area. In his book, *Empowerment Takes More than a Minute*, Blanchard states, "People already have power in their knowledge and motivation. Empowerment is releasing and focusing this power." He goes on to state that unless you create an environment that is based on trust, employees will continue to be insecure and will not feel empowered. He says that the first key to encouraging empowerment is to share accurate information with everyone. Again, his focus is to give all staff a sense of control. This is done through consistent structure and boundaries and by allowing accurate information to be shared with everyone.

To encourage autonomy in employees, he encourages the use of boundaries and structure to enhance their sense of autonomy. He stated, "Boundaries have the capacity to channel energy in a certain direction. It is like a river—if you were to take away the banks, the river would not be a river anymore. Its momentum and direction would be gone."

I couldn't say this any better. Structure and boundaries are not used for a sense of power and to control people; they are used to encourage autonomy and empowerment. Blanchard further states that the six areas in which boundaries must be created by every organization are:

1. Purpose: What business are you in?
2. Values: What are your operational guidelines?
3. Image: What is your picture of the future?
4. Goals: What, when, where, and how do you do what you do?
5. Roles: Who does what?
6. Organizational Structure and Systems: How do you support what you want to do?

The last point I want to make regarding Blanchard's book is that he encourages replacing hierarchal thinking with self-managed teams. What a concept! Organizations that remain on step one are not in position to create self-managed teams. The reason is that there is no trust. Self-managed teams will not be formed (usually) until Step Three. Health care employees need to believe in themselves and their managers. This occurs through transformational coaching. He goes on to identify the benefits of self-managed teams.

1. Increased job satisfaction
2. Attitude change from "have to" to "want to"
3. Greater employee commitment
4. Better communication between employees and management
5. More efficient decision-making process
6. Improved quality
7. Reduced operating costs
8. More profitable organization

Let's look at Marcus Buckingham and Kurt Coffman, authors of *First Break All the Rules: What the World's Greatest Managers Do Differently.* They do a wonderful job of breaking down transformational coaching. They initially place a great deal of importance on the interview and hiring process and looking for the right talent. They have found that great managers identify talent as "a recurrent pattern of thought, feeling or behavior that can be productively applied." They empha-

size the word "recurring" because it is through this consistent behavior that they will have a productive employee.

They go on to discuss that everything is easier as a result of hiring
the right individual. I can't tell you how many times nurses have told
me they do not understand why certain people were hired. They
become more confused by how much energy is spent trying to
"make" them productive.

The authors then discuss the importance of releasing each person's potential. This is done by identifying each individual's unique
personality and strengths. Doesn't this sound familiar? They state
that "One of the signs of a great manager is his ability to describe,
in detail, the unique talents of each of his or her people—what
drives each one, how each one thinks, how each builds relationships." And last, near and dear to my heart, they describe that great
managers know how to break the golden rule. "Everyone is excep-
tional and should be treated as an exception. Each employee has
their own filter, his own way of interpreting the world around him,
and therefore, each employee will demand different things of you
as her manager." This is supportive of the 4-P Personality Style and
the overall Circle of Control. When you can truly understand your
employees' Circles of Control, what makes them think, what makes
them defensive, and what motivates them, you will not only enhance the satisfaction of that employee within the hospital but you
will retain that individual for a long period of time. We could go on
and review hundreds of other management books, but I think that
these two provide you with an example of current management
techniques that support and enhance the Success Steps model.

Truth #8:

Creating Your Experience

Putting All This Together to Create a Wonderful Career and Life

You are the cause of everything that happens to you. Be careful what you cause.

—Dr. Robert Anthony

I pray that this has been a wonderful journey for you, helping you understand how special you are. You were special before you chose this profession or picked up this book. Now you have the tools to create a different experience for yourself. The choice is yours. Each day that you walk into work, you control your actions and experiences. You understand the realities and issues that are out of your control and are beginning to use the tools you have learned. Even with all the stories and techniques I have provided, some of you may still wonder if creating your ideal environment is really possible. If you have never experienced a sense of control or happiness in your life, it's no wonder.

Rest assured. This *is* possible, and you can do it. It will require some work on your part, however. Pay attention to the stories of your colleagues, practice these techniques, and start noticing the shifts occurring around—and within—you.

At the beginning of this book, I stated that this was a book about developing you, and it has been. All about you. By developing yourself and using these tools, you will find the answers to retaining our nurses and improving our shortages in the health care profession. You will reconnect with your teams and yourself in meaningful ways. The solution is not an external one but an internal one. Developing yourself and the people around you *is* the answer.

Creating Your Experience

Each of these truths and the stories behind them have given you hope that how you've experienced and perceived life can be different. I am telling you it can. You know this because you have a different sense of your self after reviewing your Circle of Control. Through the stories in this book, you can relate to the struggles, fears, and successes of the people involved. Through the use of the Success Steps model you are more confident about interacting with others and understanding how to direct that conversation, and through the use of the various guidelines for conflict management and management of teams, you have a road map on how to affect your world. Through all of this, we are missing one key variable that will further enhance your experience and your development. You are going to spend some time learning how to create an experience. What I mean to say is changing your experience in a conscious manner is a science. There are steps that you need to follow in both your thought process and what you say. These principles will assist you in creating the experience that you want, and they work in tandem with the previous truths.

Let us revisit the book *Creative Visualization* by Shakti Gawain. She describes creative visualization as a technique of using your imagination to create what you want in your life. She goes on to say that this is a natural power of our imagination and the creative energy of the universe that we constantly use to create our world. However, "Creative visualization has been used in a relatively unconscious way. Because of our own deep-seated negative concepts about life, we have automatically and unconsciously expected and imagined lack, limitation, difficulties and problems to be our lot in life. To one degree or another that is what we have created for ourselves."

I hope this sounds familiar from our earlier discussions about living life consciously and being aware of all the aspects of who you are and how that relates to your experience. Ms. Gawain is saying the same thing. She is telling you that you have the ability to create the experience that you want. She proposes that you use your imagination to create a clear image, idea, or feeling of something you wish to manifest. Then, as you continue to focus on the idea, give that positive energy until it becomes a reality.

What she is saying is that you can achieve what you imagine. Think about this: when you look at your present situation in your work world and your life and you are being honest with yourself, haven't you created this experience? Haven't you chosen how to respond and react to various individuals? Haven't you prevented yourself from imagining what a different world would be like because of the energy, work, or the impossibility in your mind of that occurring? There are four basic steps for effective creative visualization outlined in her book.

1. Setting your goal. She encourages you to make these realistic and fairly easy to attain.
2. Create a clear idea or picture. As you do this, make sure the idea is exactly what you want, and, most importantly, you need to imagine it as if you have already obtained it. I will explain the importance of this later.
3. Focus on it often. Believe that you can obtain this. Believe you can maintain it and use periods throughout the day to bring it to your mind. It can be done during times of meditation. It has to become an integral part of your thought process throughout the day, but remember, don't push too hard; just let it happen.
4. Give it positive energy. Think about your goal in a positive, supportive way. Make statements that support you obtaining this goal. Visualize yourself receiving this.

You're wondering, does this really work? How can using words and statements affirming something you want possibly make it come to you? I am telling you this works, and I'll share with you my own personal use of these four steps and what they have done for me. If you refer back to the first truth, I discussed with you how I came to write this book. I'd never written a book; I never knew how, but there was something inside of me that wanted to express a message.

In addition to this, I also wanted to return to school to begin developing people, and I didn't know what that meant. As I reviewed different schools, I wasn't sure what degree to pursue that would prepare me to develop people. I mean this very seriously. I asked different counselors at schools, "What's the best advanced degree to focus on developing people?" I got some very strange answers. I sat down and used the creative visualization steps and began to meditate, to talk to my external support systems, and to really clarify in my mind what it was I wanted to create. Through these exercises it became clear to me that I was ready to set a goal. My goal was to obtain my doctorate, focusing on the management of people and organizations. I developed a clear plan how I was going to obtain this. I envisioned myself receiving my doctorate degree. I envisioned myself consulting with other organizations with the expertise that I had developed. What I found interesting was that I found myself behaving like someone with a doctorate prior to even obtaining the degree.

I focused on this often. It became part of who I was and part of my ongoing discussions, and I began connecting myself with management and staff development organizations. Through this process I gave a great deal of positive energy to this, and I completed my degree in 2 years.

As for the book, it was a similar process. As I sat down to determine exactly what my goal would be through meditation and talking with people in my support systems, it was clear that I had expertise in health care and that the tools I had developed throughout my clinical administrative years needed to be shared. I created a clear picture of exactly what this book would look like and how it would help people. It was a daily part of my focus and energies.

Having never written before, I began to ask myself what steps I would take to make this a reality, all along truly believing that it was going to become a reality. I contacted several writers to assist me in the process, I pitched the idea to a great many publishers, and I experienced many naysayers and rejections. I was not going to let this deter me from what I wanted to create and the positive energy of envisioning what this would look like.

This isn't easy. It is very easy to begin thinking negative thoughts, to be fearful of what others are going to think about you and acknowledge the possibility of failure. Approaching life from a creative visualization approach is much more rewarding and peaceful.

Are you good enough? Some people unconsciously believe they are not. This has to change. I am going to repeat that. *This has to change.* You cannot create a new experience for yourself if the underlying belief you have about yourself is that you are not good enough. This stems from a variety of different sources, and many of you experience this today. You have reacted to the idea that you are not good enough by being less than you are and withdrawing from life. Some of you become angry and are continually argumentative with others. Some of you become controlling and attempt to replace the feelings of being out of control by controlling other parts of your lives. And some of you have faced this and have recognized that you are good enough and that whatever has occurred in your past is just that. It is in your past, and you deserve to be happy and you deserve to create an environment that is wonderful.

Tell your coworkers how wonderful they are. Send them a note. Buy them a cup of coffee. Let them know how much you appreciate them and tell them they are good enough. You will find that doing this has more of an impact on you than it does on them.

I want to mention one more aspect from the creative visualization book that I believe will help you understand how to create a new experience. Ms. Gawain says that life consists of three aspects, and these aspects make up your daily experiences. They are "being, doing and having. Being is the experience we have and we are fully focused in the present moment, the experience of being totally complete and at rest within ourselves." Doing is what it sounds like. It is the movement and activity. Having is what it sounds like as well: "It is the state of being in a relationship with other people and things in the universe."

I bring this up to help you understand how people use these aspects to create what they want in their lives. You see, these three aspects of life are interconnected. Where the concern exists is that people live their lives backwards. As Ms. Gawain puts it, they try to "*have* more things or more money in order to *do* more of what they want to, so they will *be* happier." For you truly to create the world that you want, you have to approach this in the reverse sense. You have to *be* who you are or who you visualize you're going to be, then you begin *doing* what you need to do in order to *have* what you want. Your doing part of life reflects your idea of what you are being. Does that make sense to you? Let me give you an example. I told you my goals were to obtain my doctorate and become an author, so I began doing things that reflected these two ideas. Then I started to have these things. I began reading about being an author, practiced my writing, contacted publishers and universities. My doing reflected my state of being.

When you listen to your colleagues converse about problems in your unit, in the hospital, and in their lives, listen to how they tell you this. They tell you what they *want*. For example, they want better management, they want better staffing, they want everyone to get along. Based on the principles of creative visualization, they will receive exactly that: the feeling of wanting. Then they wonder why they are unhappy. They have created the experience that they asked for. Their energies and their focus never went beyond just asking the question or making the statement of what they want.

Does this concept make sense to you? Can you understand how you can approach what you want to create at work and in your personal life? This is not just one person's idea. This is a common approach that many authors have identified. If you take a look at the book *The Power of Now* by Eckhart Tolle (1997), there is an entire chapter called "Moving Deeply into the Now." His premise is that in the now or the "being," there is no anxiety. Anxiety cannot exist in this state. Where anxiety exists is through living in the past or in the future. We can become so preoccupied with what we've done wrong and what is going to happen to us that we miss out on living in the power of now. This is his emphasis, and it supports creative visualization and the previous truths on using those tools in the moment. We discussed this in truth seven when we reviewed breathing techniques. The point of breathing and deep relaxation exercises, along with meditation, is to place yourself in the present, the now.

In addition to using these principles, consider how you can apply them in all aspects of your life. What I am trying to say here is that you will use these principles in all aspects of your life. Because you have learned the principles from each of the eight truths, you will inevitably approach each relationship in your life differently. You will perceive stress and the external world in a different manner as well, so take a moment and not only spend time evaluating your work place relationships, but look at your personal relationships too.

I shared with you stories of my personal relationship with my wife. It is a topic that I will elaborate on in future books, but for your own sense of self and happiness in life, I encourage you to apply these principles to your world outside of work.

More specifically, use the Control Reaction Map when you are interacting in personal relationships. Attempt to understand the personality styles of others with whom you share your life. Recognize that they do not process or approach the world the way that you do, and when you become frustrated and angry and are feeling out of control, stop the interaction before your acting-out behavior worsens the situation.

I have always said that couples should wake up each day and ask the question, "How can I help you be in control today?" Many of the disagreements would dissipate.

Before I end this book, I want to leave you with one more story, the one that has been one of my main inspirations in writing this book. It helped me understand and confirm the principles I have shared with you in a way that even surprised me. I hope it has an impact on you.

It was a cold day in October, and I had just returned from Boston where I was working with a hospital that was extremely defensive about change and was struggling with the idea of using my principles. It had been a grueling 3 days, and I usually don't like to do more than one training session in a week. Because this was a hospital in my hometown and close to my work, I felt comfortable providing training, even though my energy and enthusiasm were not at their highest levels. I knew the director from previous meetings and was encouraged by her attitude and professionalism.

All her staff respected Diane. She prided herself on her steady leadership and her dedication to the science of nursing. She had received many awards throughout her 22-year nursing career. Diane was a tall and slender woman, which added to her confident appearance. Nothing seemed to fluster her, and she was always a rock to her peers and staff. She described to me a time in which a major restructuring had occurred that could have potentially affected her job and her staff. With all of her staff concerned about their futures and hers as well, she lived up to her perception by immediately bringing them all together and reassuring them. Without knowing that everything was going to be all right for her or for them or that her life was not going to be affected, she provided a sense of reassurance to put her staff at ease.

Diane was dedicated to her job and her staff, often arriving early in the morning and then not leaving until late. What was odd is that no one really knew who Diane was outside of work. As I said earlier, I had the privilege of meeting Diane when I was working in Grand Rapids, Michigan. I was equally impressed with her presence and her articulation. There was no indication during my training with her that there were any issues. In fact, it was the opposite. I had never met anybody who adapted so well to the principles I was teaching and made them applicable to her work and life. She understood the Success Steps model and, one could say was a poster child for the use of these principles. She was the first one to support my work to her peers, her staff, and administration. I felt that she was my big-gest fan during those training days.

This is what makes the story so interesting. You see, I spend a great deal of energy teaching people to think differently, to experi-ence a new outcome. Diane was already there. She was demon-strating my principles and modeling them to her staff. What I did not do is really understand her motivation. I did not ask why she had chosen this path. Who cares, right? She was doing all the right things. Why should I care how and why she was there? She was just there.

Diane taught me a valuable lesson that day. She taught me that just because you may be practicing these principles, you could still be living your life unconsciously, and this is exactly what was occur-ring with Diane.

After completing the training, I received a note from one of the staff, which was not unusual. Many people approach me after I speak to talk individually. What was different about this note was that it was not about them. All the note said was, "Please talk with Diane; we are all worried about her."

I was caught off guard and was not sure what to do. I paused for a moment and found myself looking around the room to see if I could determine who wrote the note. I couldn't. By the time I looked up, most people had left, but before I could think any longer, someone had tapped me on the shoulder. It was Diane.

I must have had a startled look on my face because she asked me what was wrong. I told her I was fine and was just reviewing the training in my mind, but I couldn't get the note out of my thoughts. As I was collecting my papers, I decided to approach Diane. When I asked if we could speak, she warmly said yes. I assumed she was thinking we were going to speak about her staff and the training.

I asked her how she was doing. Without hesitation, in the same professional manner as always, she said she was great. She imme-diately began speaking about the challenges with work. I inter-rupted her and repeated my question. "How are *you* doing?" She looked at me puzzled as if I had not understood her answer. She asked, "What do you mean?" I repeated myself slowly. "Diane, I want to know how you are doing." The pause seemed dramatic. It was the first time I saw Diane without an answer. From the looks of it, I think it surprised her as well. She attempted to answer my ques-tion but struggled completing a sentence. I placed my hand on her arm and told her that her staff was worried about her.

Her eyes began to tear up and she quickly attempted to look away from me. I told her it was all right; she did not have to hold back from me. I told her it was safe. Diane began to cry and reached out to give me a hug. Her crying grew louder as I told her to let it go. For over 5 minutes, Diane cried. I did not say much, just encouraged her to let it out. As she began to compose herself, I asked her if we could talk about this, but she was hesitant. She told me she had kept things in so long that she did not know if she could let them out.

After I encouraged her, she began to tell me things about her life that no one else knew. She told me she was a phony. She felt that every day she was pretending. She said, "The reason I appear to have it all together is to hide from people how messed up my life is. Work is the one place I can create a different world. That is why I do not interact with anyone outside of work and have clear boundaries with my staff. They see it as being professional, and I see it as protection."

Then it hit me. Diane was right. Whatever was taking place in her life, it was making her feel out of control. The only way she could feel in control was to create a world where she was seen as a consummate professional. I asked if she would be willing to tell me how she arrived at this position. She hesitated but had a sense of trust with me. She went on to tell me that she had been in an abusive marriage for 13 years. She cynically told me it was not physical, just verbal (as if that was different or less severe). She went on to describe how for those 13 years she lived in a controlling house with a husband who managed all the finances and increasingly questioned her time out of the home. She noticed a severe change in his behavior when she finished her master's degree in nursing. After that, he began to drink more and verbally put her down. Earlier in their marriage the abuse seem to occur only in their home. Towards the end, it occurred in public as well.

At his company Christmas party, he had too much to drink. He began telling everyone that since his wife finished her master's, she was "too damn smart" for him. He began describing to others how stupid she was when it came to common sense activities at home. When they returned home that evening, she confronted him and he responded by saying, "Since you have finished your degree, you only care about work. You stink as a mother, and you're a worse wife."

Diane then said, "I haven't told anyone that story before." She paused. "I left him after that evening. It took me 13 years to do it."

However, it was too late. The damage was done. I asked her, "Is that when you decided to create this perfect world?" She said yes. "My staff always wonders why I never socialize with them or talk about my personal life. I cannot let the secret out! But it feels good to be honest. I am slowly believing that I am a good person. Intellectually, I know that I am, but some days I can't believe it."

I asked her if we could begin again with the Success Steps techniques now that she was being honest. She agreed. She was a processor and a peacemaker. Her most important self-worth issues centered on being a role model for other nurses and a mom to her two grown daughters. She told me she had external support systems but no one with whom she had shared this information.

She understood her abusive relationship had led her to feel out of control. Unlike most people who feel out of control, Diane responded by creating a positive controlling environment. She acted out by avoiding this issue with her husband and others. What she was creating was a nonexistent relationship. Consciously and unconsciously, she began to understand this and got a divorce, but she never spent time to understand these dynamics to reconnect with herself.

Closing:

Where Do We Go From Here?

Putting It All Together

It is wise to direct your anger towards problems—
not people; to focus your energies on answers—not excuses.

—William Arthur Ward

You are the future of nursing. In our profession, we must begin training our nurses and health professionals in a different manner. It can no longer be business as usual. The research, and your own personal experiences, are proof that "business as usual" doesn't work. There needs to be a shift in consciousness.

The practice of nursing (as many other health care professions) is based on a set of scientific principles and evidence-based practice patterns. This is important and critical to the advancement of these professions. However, we need to include in our scientific foundation the principles of emotional health and connection. The ideals encapsulated in these principles need to be mandatory for all health care employees. Without them, careers of employees and lives of patients and families will be impacted.

Steve Adubato, author of *Speak from the Heart,* discussed the communication challenge, in many ways, as the most important aspect of delivering superior health care. He goes on to say that the best technology and research has its place, but health care is largely about human interaction between patients who are sick and the professionals who are expected to have all the answers but clearly don't.

I could not have articulated this any better. Much of our work is based on human interactions. We need to understand and instruct students in the science of human interaction. Without this focus, we not only place new nurses at a disadvantage, we potentially place ourselves in a position of not managing stress and conflict in a professional and productive manner.

We need to establish a curriculum in our schools that includes the principles for developing and managing teams, understanding various personality styles, and ways to communicate effectively with patients and families. Understanding communication patterns at all levels is the one technique that can make or break your team. Mastering this can create a safe and clinically effective environment, as well as create a sense of fulfillment in your own life wherever you may work. You know from reading this book that these principles are applicable in all aspects of your life. In addition to using these principles and tools at work, consider how you can apply them in all aspects of your life.

Recruiting and Job Satisfaction

I highly encourage you to review the Advisory Board Company's series, "Nurse Retention and Job Satisfaction." These articles provide excellent insight on how to obtain and retain nurses. I want to review a few of their principles that support the idea of where we are going to go from here and on what our attention needs to focus.

According to the Advisory Board Company's manuscript, "Nursing's Next Generation: Best Practice for Attracting, Training and Retaining New Graduates," there are three major categories to focus on enhancing the experience of the next generation of nurses and recruiting top talent.

1. Offer competitive compensation.
2. Offer scheduling options.
3. Partner with nursing schools.

Offer Competitive Compensation

The advisory board reviewed three individual practices with the purpose of ensuring that competitive compensation is offered to new recruits. The first one is to make sure that there is a comprehensive evaluation of offers. Make sure each candidate understands exactly what's included in a pay and benefits package. So often there is a focus on an hourly rate and little emphasis on shift differentials and other benefits.

Market-based compensation encourages an understanding of an area's top salaries and ensures you are within the range of those top salaries. You have all seen the back-and-forth salary increases of various hospitals as they compete for the highest hourly wage for nurses. It is important to be in the appropriate range.

The last practice pattern discussed was pay for performance. This is a fairly new approach for hospitals, looking at compensation based on actual nursing performance rather than just tenure or experience. This can be attractive to new graduates who feel they can control their own pace of growth (and pay) based on their efforts and progress.

Scheduling Options

We reviewed in truth one the importance that nurses place on the flexibility of their schedules. This is by far one of the most important aspects of retaining nurses throughout the country. It is not a complicated approach.

Self-scheduling has been widely popular with many nursing groups. It makes sense. We talked about having a sense of control of your workplace, which puts you in a position to feel in control. Self-scheduling does that. There are a variety of different types of self-scheduling options out there, but the fundamental consistency among all of them is there has to be a set of guidelines individuals must follow, i.e., certain weekends must be worked, holidays must be rotated, and everyone must work a mix of evenings and nights.

Where it becomes difficult is when managers and directors have brought people in on set schedules and then moved to a self-scheduling model, leaving few options for the remaining staff. I encourage you to sit down with the team, develop a scheduling group, and identify a set of principles that everyone can support. The mistake that is made is that people jump into doing the actual schedule without these principles. As a result, people become frustrated and angry and do not benefit from the use of self-scheduling.

One other popular option that is occurring is the establishment of 9-month contracts. Certain hospitals and health care institutions have found that their census decreases in the summertime and have offered some nurses 9-month contracts. You can understand the popularity of this for those who have children who are out of school during the summertime. I am not saying that it would fit into your organization, but it is well worth evaluating.

Partnering with Nursing Schools

A variety of different initiatives have been identified in partnering with nursing schools. These initiatives ensure that nursing education is aligned with nursing practice patterns in your hospital to develop student nursing internships. This enhances their clinical skills and gives them a sense of safety and security as they develop these new skills.

I am concerned about our new nurses because many do not have the tools to manage stress and are more likely to burn out. Specifically, these nurses fit the personality profile outlined in truth six. Anything that can be done to help decrease their stress level and enhance their sense of safety through connection with specific mentors will be helpful.

These are just a few ideas that we can pursue as we identify where we are going from here with regard to our new nursing graduates. The use of the Success Steps model and the Control Reaction Map will provide you with more than enough guidance to ensure that somebody new in your organization feels welcomed and cared for.

Putting All This Together

I want this last section to be a synopsis of the work that you did for the first three truths. This approach will allow you to review the answers you gave. Let's begin.

Understanding Your Reality

As we have identified, the realities you deal with everyday at work impact your life. You may perceive some of these realities as stressors. Others you may identify as positive experiences while some have little to no impact on you.

Regardless of what category these realities are in, it is important for you to be conscious of them. For those realities that you have identified as stressors it is important to categorize which ones you can impact and which ones are out of your control. Just completing the task of listing these stressors will provide you with a sense of comfort.

Below is a list (1–10) that I would like you to complete. Please identify your perceived stressors that impact your daily work life, 1 being the most severe and 10 being the least.

1.

2.

3.

4.

5.

6.

7.

8.

9.

10.

Next to each stressor place a checkmark for those that you have direct control, two checkmarks for those that you have partial control, and an "X" next to the stressors that are completely out of your control.

Look at your top ten and the corresponding marks. Have you identified what is really in your control? If it is not in your control, let it go! Don't keep giving energy to these areas. Place your efforts into the stressors you can impact. Go ahead start to make a plan to impact these stressors.

Let's review your personal Circle of Control.

Look at your Circle of Control and make sure you are comfortable with the picture of who you are. Now what I want you to do is evaluate your Circle of Control and determine if there is a correlation between it and the stressor that you have identified. For example, if the number one stressor that you have identified in your workplace is nonsupportive and at times incompetent staff and you have a 4-P Personality Style as a processor, what does this tell you?

YOUR 4-P PERSONALITY STYLE:

Your specific self-worth list (You can copy your list from Truth #2, page 34):

Priority List	Evidence
1.	
2.	
3.	
4.	
5.	

It is important to understand how your perception of these individuals may be more critical as a result of your personality style. This is how I want you to use this tool as it relates to your stress.

Look at your specific self-worth. Is there any area that you identified that is of utmost importance to you and, concurrently, is an issue as a high area of stress in your life? For example, if your number one specific self-worth goal is to be a loving and caring mother and your number one stressor is your inflexible schedule, which is not allowing you to spend more time at home, what does this tell you? I want you to make these connections and have a conscious understanding of how all these are connected together. To steal a phrase, from Stephen Covey, "Begin with the end in mind."

I leave you with this phrase because I think of it as the most important point for you to remember. Each of these truths builds on the others. They provide you with a human interaction model that you have not experienced before. Your success in the workplace and, more importantly, in your life will be based on your ability to interact and to find a sense of peace and joy in what you do.

By beginning with the end in mind, you have an understanding of what you want to create. You can visualize what this end should look like and begin to follow the path in that direction.

I hope these truths and these tools provide you a sense of confidence to achieve your dreams. God bless you.

REFERENCES

Abrams, M. R., Numerof, R. E., & Ott, B. (2004). Building a nursing leadership infrastructure. *Nurse Leader*, Feb, 33–37.

Adams, B. (1998). *Managing people: Lead your staff to peak performance*. Avon, MA: Streetwise Publication.

Adubato, S. (2002). *Speak from the heart*. New York: The Free Press.

Advisory Board. (2000). *The nurse perspective: Drivers of nurse job satisfaction and turnover*. Washington, DC: Author.

Advisory Board. (2002). *Nurses next generation: Best practices for attracting, training and retaining new graduates*. Washington, DC: Author.

Belitz, C., & Lundstrom, M. (1998). *The power of flow: Practical ways to transform your life with meaningful coincidence*. New York: Three Rivers Press.

Blanchard, K. (2001). *Empowerment takes more than a minute*. San Francisco: Berret-Kochler Publishers.

Borda, R. G., & Norman, I. (1997). Factors influencing turnover and absence of nurses: A research review. *International Journal of Nursing Studies*, 34(6), 385–394.

Buck, E. A., & Loveland Cook, C. A. (1999). Caring for yourself during times of organizational change. *Seminars for Nurse Managers*, 7(3), 141–148.

Buckingham, M., & Coffman, K. (1999). *First break all the rules: What the world's greatest managers do differently*. New York: Simon and Schuster.

Bush, J. P. (1988). Job satisfaction, powerlessness, and loss of control. *Western Journal of Nursing Research*, 10(7), 8–431.

Butler, J., & Parsons, R. (1989). Hospital perception of job satisfaction. *Nursing Management*, 20(8), 45–48.

Carlson-Catalano, J. (1990). Hospital nurse experiences. In L. Gasporis & J. Swirsky (Eds.), *Nurse Abuse: Its Impact and Resolution* (pp. 125–174). New York: Power Publications.

Chansarkar, B., Maylor, U., & Newman, K. (2001). The nurse retention, quality of care and patient satisfaction chain. *International Journal of Healthcare Quality Assurance*, 14(2), 57–68.

Cohen, S. (2004). Leadership standards: No room for doubt. *Nursing Management*, 35(8), 10, 14.

Couture, R. T., & Kivisto, J. (1997). Stress management for nurses: Controlling the whirlwind. *Nursing Forum*, 32(1), 25–33.

Cullen, A. (1995). Burnout: Why do we blame the nurse? *American Journal of Nursing*, 95(11), 22–27.

Davidhizar, R., Eshleman, J., & Shearer, R. (1999). Praise that matters. *Seminars for Nurse Managers*, 7(2), 86–89.

Davies, C. (1995). *Gender and the professional predicament in nursing*. Philadelphia: Open University Press.

Dimitrius, J. (1999). *How to understand people and predict their behavior anytime, anyplace*. New York: Ballantine.

Droppleman, P., & Thomas, S. (1997). Channeling nurses' anger into positive interventions. *Nursing Forum*, 32(2), 13–21.

Erickson, J.I., & Nevidjon, B. (2001). The nursing shortage: Solutions for the short and long term. *Online Journal of Issues in Nursing*, 6(1), 1–12.

Fey, M., & Miltner, R. (2000). A competency-based orientation program for new graduate nurses. *Journal of Nursing Administration*, 30(3), 126–132.

Frings-Dresen, M. H. W., Sluiter, J. K., van Saane, N., & Verbeek, J. H. A. N. (2003). Reliability and validity of instruments measuring job satisfaction: A systematic review. *Occupational Medicine*, 53, 191–200.

Gawain, S. (1995). *Creative visualization*. Novato, CA: Publishers Group West.

Helge, D. (2001). Turning workplace anger and anxiety into peak performance: Strategies for enhancing employee health and productivity. *American Association of Occupational Health Nurses Journal*, 49(8), 399–406.

Hillhouse, J., & Adler, C. (in press). Investigating unique patterns of stress-related symptomatology in hospital staff nurses: Results of a cluster analysis. *Social Science and Medicine*.

Johnston, C. L. (1997). Changing care patterns and registered nurse job satisfaction. *Holistic Nursing Practice*, 3, 69–77.

Jones, W. J. (2002). Staffing shortages: How did we get here? *Social Science & Medicine*, 8(6), 18–23.

Joni, S. A. (2004). The geography of trust. *Harvard Business Review*, March, 82–88.

Kalisch, B., & Kalisch, P. (1977). An analysis of the sources of physician-nurse conflict. *Journal of Nursing Administration, 7*(1), 51–57.

Kirkhart, K. (1996). Caregiving and burnout: Are you at risk? *Generations*, Winter, 6–8.

Langemo, D. K. (1990). Inpact of work stress on female nurse educators. *Image Journal of Nursing, 22*(3), 159–162.

Malloch, K., & Porter-O'Grady, T. (2002). *Quantum leadership: A textbook of new leadership.* Sudbury, MA: Jones and Bartlett Publishers.

Manderino, M., & Berkey, N. (1995). Verbal abuse of staff nurses by physicians. *Image, 27*, 244.

Manion, J. (2004). Nurture a culture of retention. *Nursing Management, 35*(4), 29–39.

McKenna, H. (1998). Editorials: The professional cleansing of nurses. *British Medical Journal, 317*, 1403–1404.

Minchington, J. (1993). *Maximum self-esteem: The handbook for reclaiming your sense of self-worth.* Banzant, MO: Arnford House Publishers.

Muff, J. (1982). *Women's issues in nursing: Socialization, sexism and stereotyping.* Prospect Heights, IL: Waveland Press.

Nursing Executive Center. (2000). *Reversing the flight of talent: Executive briefing.* Washington, DC: The Advisory Board Company.

O'Hara, V. (1995). *Wellness 9 to 5: Managing stress at work.* New York: MJF Publishing.

Ponterdolph, M., & Toscano, P. (1998). The personality to buffer burnout. *Nursing Management, 29*(8), 1–2.

Rodgers, J. A. (1982). Women and the fear of being envied. *Nursing Outlook, 30*, 344–347.

Schwab, L. (1996). Individual hardiness in staff satisfaction. *Nursing Economics, 14*(3), 171–173.

Short, J. D. (1997). Psychological effects of stress from restructuring and reorganization. *American Association of Occupational Health Nurses Journal, 45*(11), 597–604.

Smith, G., & Seccumbe, I. (1998). *Changing times: A survey of registered nurses in 1998.* Report 351, Institute for Employment Studies, Brighton, England.

Stokols, D. (1992). Conflict-prone and conflict-resistant organizations. In H. Friedmann (Ed.), *Hostility, coping and health* (pp. 65–76). Washington, DC: American Psychological Association.

Tolle, E. (1997). *The power of now.* Nevada, CA: Namaste Publishing.

Waite, R., Buchan, J., & Thomas, J. (1989). *Nurses in and out of work.* Institute of Manpower Studies, Brighton, England.

Walsch, N. D. (1997). *Conversations with god: An uncommon dialogue.* Charlottesville, VA: Hampton Roads Publishing Company, Inc.

Walsch, N. D. (2004). *Tomorrow's god: Our greatest spiritual challenge.* New York: Atria Books.